Pre-publication Praise for *Secrets...*

"*The Secrets of Medical Decision Making* is an important book. It should be read by everyone, because all of us are sometimes in need of medical care. It is an eye-opener, a call to arms and a guide."
—Robert Rich, Ph.D., MAPS, AASH,
author of *Cancer: A Personal Challenge*

"Dr. Reznik candidly exposes the conflicting interests inherent in contemporary medical practice. He encourages patients and their family members to be knowledgeable and pro-active healthcare consumers by asking questions, evaluating research, trusting personal preferences, and understanding the limitations of modern medicine. This empowering and insightful book is a must read for healthcare professionals and the patients they treat." —Beth Maureen Gray, R.N., B.S.

"*The Secrets of Medical Decision Making* awakens the reader rather quickly with startling revelations about the lack of seriousness the health care industry has towards a society of wellness. Patients in today's society resemble an assembly line as they are pushed through a healthcare system that seeks to serve and protect the medical industry at the expense of the patient's health, safety, and welfare. If this book at least motivates its readers to become more involved in medical decision making when seeking treatment, it will have succeeded as a critically needed public service."
—Rev. James W. Clifton, Ph.D., LCSW

"This is a profound book for the layman. Many times a doctor never levels with their patients because the doctor wants to spare us the pain of dealing with the illness or disease. I know, from personal experience, I'm more hurt and suspicious of my doctor when they behave this way rather than telling me plainly. I recommend *The Secrets of Medical Decision Making* to all patients interested in their health and keeping healthy."
—Lillian Cauldwell

The Secrets of Medical Decision Making:

How to Avoid Becoming
a Victim of the Health Care Machine

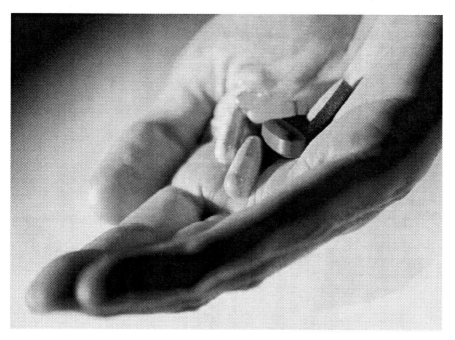

By
Oleg I. Reznik, M.D.

Foreword by
Colin P. Kopes-Kerr, MD, JD, MPH

The Secrets of Medical Decision Making: How to Avoid Becoming a Victim of the Health Care Machine.

First Edition: January 2006

Library of Congress Cataloging-in-Publication Data

Reznik, Oleg I.
   The secrets of medical decision making : how to avoid becoming a victim of the health care machine / by Oleg I. Reznik ; foreword by Colin P. Kopes-Kerr.-- 1st ed.
      p. cm.
   Includes bibliographical references and index.
   ISBN-13: 978-1-932690-16-3 (case laminate : alk. paper)
   ISBN-10: 1-932690-16-6 (case laminate : alk. paper)
   ISBN-13: 978-1-932690-17-0 (trade paper : alk. paper)
   ISBN-10: 1-932690-17-4 (trade paper : alk. paper)
   1. Patient participation. 2. Medical care--Decision making. 3. Physician and patient. I. Title.
R727.42.R49 2006
610.69'6--dc22
                              2005019931

Distributed by:
Baker & Taylor, Ingram Book Group

Published by:
Loving Healing Press
5145 Pontiac Trail
Ann Arbor, MI 48105
USA

http://www.LovingHealing.com or
info@LovingHealing.com
Fax +1 734 663 6861

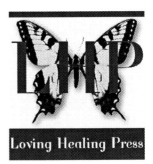

Loving Healing Press

To Mathilde.

About the Author

Oleg I. Reznik, M.D is a Board Certified Family Physician working at the Willamette Family Medical Center and in private practice, on staff at Salem Memorial Hospital, Salem, OR.

Family Medicine Residency Program at State University of New York (SUNY) Stony Brook, Stony Brook, NY 2000-2003;

MD degree *cum laude* at SUNY Downstate, Brooklyn, NY 1996-2000;

Bachelor's degree in Neuroscience *cum laude* at New York University, New York, NY 1991-1995;

Table of Contents

Table of Figures

Acknowledgments

I would like to express my appreciation to Dr. Kopes-Kerr for his brilliant professional newsletters, which were the source of a great deal of the supporting material used in this book; for his inspiring character, and for writing a foreword to this book.

I would like to thank Dr. Bob Rich for his invaluable help in editing this book. During this journey together I had the privilege of contributing to his book *CANCER: A Personal Challenge*, which is an invaluable resource for cancer sufferers and their families.

I would like to thank the Trustees of Dartmouth College, who have given their permission to use the wealth of information concentrated in The Dartmouth Atlas of Health Care, with excerpts and diagrams, free of charge.

Foreword
by Colin P Kopes–Kerr, MD, JD, MPH

Where has Marcus Welby, MD, gone—that prime-time hero of the 1969 TV medical drama starring actor Robert Young? We really need him now. Sadly, this image of a gentle friend and neighbor to his patients, who relied more on his caring and belonging to his community than upon bio-engineered pharmaceuticals and high-resolution computerized imaging techniques, is nowhere to be found in the early 21st century. This is disappointing, even to physicians, many of whom entered the non-specialized area of primary care with this gratifying model very fresh in their minds. What happened to the home town physicians who based their diagnoses and treatments on personal knowledge of patients and their context? They have quietly disappeared through retirement or disillusion with the social changes (of which there are many—managed care, malpractice crises, federal regulation, etc.) that have transformed medicine. They have not been replaced.

Everything in medicine has changed. The social and cultural context in which patients live has changed dramatically—with less job security, higher unemployment, less insurance coverage, higher deductibles, and a pervasive mistrust of civic leaders. US society now tolerates a clear and widespread social division between the medical "haves" (those with good health insurance) and the "have nots" (those without medical insurance). Both groups have profound medical problems, but they are very different. Medical education now limits the vision of "family doctors" by recruiting mostly those who are destined to be specialists wielding high-technology diagnostic devices or state-of-the-art intrusions into the body for various repairs. The content of medical education has become highly research-based, specialist-oriented, and focuses almost exclusively on secondary prevention (what to do after a disease has already become manifest, and directed only towards those with good health insurance), rather than on the truly life-saving, life-prolonging strategies that comprise primary prevention (steps to avoid the disease in the first place). Conveniently forgotten is the fact that improvements in sanitary conditions are responsible for most of the longevity we have achieved, and that the most impressive, cost-effective, and high-yield medical interventions are still simple things like diet, exercise, vitamins, and aspirin.

The landscape for physicians to find opportunities to practice has been radically altered by governmental and legal constraints. The only physicians who will be financially rewarded are those who seek to deliver high-margin services to the well-to-do (meaning at a minimum those with good health insurance), in popular living centers where new physicians are least needed. They will generally work for large, impersonal organizations that are rich enough to manage legal risk, monitor compliance with all applicable local, state, and federal regulatory constraints, insure aggressive risk management practices and maintain adequate malpractice coverage in order to insure the ability of the enterprise to continue participating in the potential profits of medical practice. Patients have to turn to relatively soulless, mega-corporate enterprises, being conducted by warring behemoths—large insurance companies (Aetna, US Health, United, etc.), pharmaceutical drug companies (Pfizer, Merck, Lilly, etc.), medical and biotechnology engineering companies (GE, Johnson & Johnson, Hewlet Packard, Genentech, Medtronic, Guidant, etc.), and very successful political lobbies for all these groups plus additional special interest groups like AARP and the Trial Lawyers Association. This landscape should be readily recognizable to all of us; some part of it gets a new headline everyday. Conspicuously absent from the widespread media coverage of the modern American health miracle is a concern for the "average" citizen's healthcare experience or the patient outcome that really matters—the number of preventable years-of-life-lost. We should urgently be asking, "Where do we fit in?" as both patients and physicians. Survival is not particularly easy in this world, but it can be graceful.

This is the starting point for Dr. Oleg Reznik's new book, *The Secrets of Medical Decision Making: How to Avoid Becoming a Victim of the Health Care Machine*. Dr. Reznik is a recently trained (at a prestigious northeastern university hospital) physician, now in the small-town practice of Family Medicine in the US Northwest; he has had previous careers as a nurse and as a patient. He knows what he is talking about. While there are numerous recent books that critique various parts of the current health care in the US; they focus on the major external forces coming to bear on the system— pharmaceutical industry, the malpractice crisis, the regulatory environment, the biotechnology revolution, the failure of health insurance, and many more. Dr. Reznik's book is different. He elucidates the interior psychodynamic processes that go on in both physicians and patients that have made these outside forces so incredibly and regrettably successful. He tries to demonstrate that the only way to get effective health care is to get inside the heads of the individuals who operate the system, the doctors and the patients, and find out how they think, and, in fact, how they make the decisions they do. This is both a challenging and a hugely rewarding process. It turns out that neither group is making logical decisions, if you define "logical" as meaning rationally related to their best outcome. It is worth spending some time with an exploration of "Why not?"

On the physician side you find the paradoxical result that the elaborately specialized, research-based, system of educating physicians is actually inimical to original, creative, and individualized problem solving. Medical students are being taught that some technical marvel or pending drug development is the answer to all medical problems, they are led to believe that the root of all problems is a biochemical or anatomical problem amenable to biotechnology or surgery. They are taught that "good medicine" does not involve creativity, or relationship-oriented compromises with technical standards, but that it consists merely of following rules, guidelines, "care maps," and "standards of care." All of these plunge the patient into ever-increasing medical testing and medical interventions. The role of the generalist physician is only to refer the patient to the appropriate technician (i.e., specialist). Of course, no status-conscious student wants to go into the generalist field; the few Marcus-Welby-minded exceptions are usually relatively quickly disillusioned by low-status, low-income, or mere boredom. All of this represents a derangement. The history of medicine, starting with Hippocrates, has taught that it is the person who has the illness, who defines what is needed for care and how a "successful" treatment should evolve. The modern limited, technological vision of medicine is a temporary aberration, and an enormous act of hubris by corporate, governmental, and medical leaders.

This book is not just for patients. It is appropriately dedicated to physicians as well. It reminds them of the contemporary medical training process and how it acts on common patient examples. It will not take much self-reflection for most physicians to recognize how confined they are within the modern "medical box" that Dr. Reznik describes—confined by the financial and time pressure of modern organization of heath care delivery, the prevailing, mechanistic model of human illness and disease, the technology- and pharmaceutical-oriented bias of most contemporary medical "expert" guidelines for care, and finally by the feeling of devastating financial vulnerability for a bad outcome, should they practice anything but main-stream care. How else to explain why our national healthcare expert and consensus guidelines are so much stricter, and our costs so much greater than any other industrialized country, without anything better in the way of results to show for it? Physicians need to acknowledge, even though they are not responsible for the system, that they do, in fact, as Dr. Reznik points out, have "a vested interest in patients undergoing all of the recommended screening procedures [and that] fear and convenience drive doctors to try to impose the guidelines upon their patients, without verifying whether the recommendations are really good for those patients." The traditional elements associated with our vision of a 'family doctor' have taken a remote back seat to these forces. Gone are the most valuable aspects of real caring, as Dr. Reznik puts it—"genuine compassion, a desire to do what is in the patient's absolute best interest, and the courage to take necessary risks." For most physicians, the question of why don't they slow down, perform fewer tests, and spend more time with their patients presents a persistent, painful dilemma. How do we get back to what we were after in the first place? Dr. Reznik offers some answers. The first element required is simply courage—the courage to stand apart and just to be willing to think for oneself about what a patient needs, because we know all the social, financial, emotional, and spiritual forces acting upon her better than any other expert in the whole medical system. "It is far more comfortable for a general practitioner to send a patient for multiple studies and to multiple specialists than trying to shoulder the responsibility alone." The answer to this dilemma is a frank discussion with patients, acknowledging the limits of both the research base of modern medicine and the way in which it has been implemented in practice, and honest education about our very limited ability to produce spectacular results. We must first disclose to patients that we are not omnipotent in the realm of health and that the "health care machine" lacks any real cure for most disease, despite the glamour and much publicized stories of a few exceptions. This is a very humbling role for physicians. It requires a great deal of courage.

In trying to get into the mind of patients, Dr. Reznik's only assumption is: "When we enter the system as patients, we are simply hoping that a physician will take good care of us." What he shows us, in some harrowing detail, are the steps by which this simple, basic human motive gets betrayed by the very same system of healthcare that we are so proud of in the U.S.—the fabled heart-lung transplants, cancer cures, and the unparalleled array of advanced technology to throw at any problem, i.e., "the health care machine." It is a system that all of the players—both patients and physicians—desperately want to believe in. They all need to take note and listen to Dr. Reznik's description of how and why it is not working. He vividly supports his hard-earned conclusion with poignant and persuasive examples from real patients' lives. He also professes his other major assumption, that "emotional, mental, social, moral, and spiritual aspects of a human being may be fundamental in developing and maintaining health."

Dr. Reznik's account is so specially valuable because it reveals the inner workings of a physician's mind, not only to the physician who is capable of self-reflection, but to the patient as well, so that he or she can remove the halo from their personal physician and allow him or her to be a mere human, much like oneself, again. He cites numerous examples of how patients and families make their medical decisions, and, specifically, of how they often lose track of their original goal of the longest life possible with the greatest degree of comfort, and become constrained by the four corners of the physician's 'medical box' and by their own need to impute "omnipotence" either to their doctor, or even where there is obvious contrary evidence to this, to the "health care machine." The critical impact of Dr. Reznik's work will lie in enabling both sides of the ordinary medical encounter to see and understand how their routine, well-intended, very human behaviors conspire together to produce a result that achieves neither quality life nor quality healthcare. Change can only come from enlightened joint participation in the process. The case examples that Dr. Reznik provides are real, timely, typical, and should in their broad outlines be familiar to everyone. Their message is coherent, and compelling. Blind or automatic deference to the "health care machine" is only the pursuit of an illusion, which directly results in more suffering, not less. Achievable health lies far more in consciously living one's own life, pursuant to one's own values, and in partnering with a supportive advisor, who has no bias other than to see that you get as much of your self-defined healthcare needs met as possible. "Be your own authority, or be someone else's agenda"—is as true for the physician as it is for the patient. For both more courage and more autonomy is prescribed.

Dr. Reznik has the uncommon wisdom not to label various persons and pressures as merely "evil." In every case they represent what started off as a good intention, but which has, through very understandable human failings, gone wrong. The process is always rational, understandable, and sympathetic; it is just flawed. He reminds us that each of us have numerous instances of similar failings in our own history. We need to start out in empathy and compassion and respond to the system in ways that foster respect and civility. But the key is to start with a staunch and immutable respect for yourself and confidence in your ability to determine your own needs.

In addition to painting a detailed portrait of the current health care delivery interface, Dr. Reznik has a rich supply of very practical, common sense tips. A good physician has to overcome approval seeking and prospectively manage appropriate expectations. Physicians can manage their legal fears by realizing that "lawsuits are not about bad outcomes. They are not about bad relationships. They are about expectations." The higher we set patients' level of expectations for outcomes, the greater the legal risk we assume. The most effective way to mitigate this is by educating patients and partnering with them in the pursuit of *their* objectives. This requires adapting medical knowledge to specific consumer needs. A physician should, for example, be able to tell a patient, in ordinary lay language, whether they are at high- or low-risk for any condition that is the target of a screening program, before advising his patient to participate. It is also appropriate to tell your patient honestly whether it is a screening program that you participate in yourself.

"When nothing seems like a good option, it is better to do nothing, than to rush in"—should be a mantra for both physicians and patients.

Dr. Reznik tells patients to be prepared to make decisions in the face of uncertainty because the medical system is simply unable to provide certainty. "The patient," is the one, however, who "has to take the initiative about a decision to stop." Often all that is needed is for her to give the physician permission to stop the pursuit of certainty. "Just stopping and accepting some uncertainty and some possibility of disease and death will almost always save one from additional unnecessary suffering." As for testing, he says, "If a physician in the U.S. did not offer it himself, you probably do not need it." In treatment of a medical condition, patients should realize that, "if the doctor who offers you the treatment cannot give you the likelihood of benefit, it is best not to proceed with the treatment." "Do not go along with what you are asked to do just to be nice to your doctor." "…If you feel you're being convinced, sold, or pressured—[the] doctor's motives are probably questionable. When being pressured, do not give in." Patients would do well to heed his advice, "[I]f a doctor makes you feel afraid, recognize it as a signal not to follow his advice, and smile." Patients should also listen to Dr. Reznik when he shows how too much of a 'good thing'—health insurance—can lead to some very bad results; in particular, stay away from "routine" tests. "It is better for a patient not to undergo a screening test at all rather then undergoing one without understanding it." In one of his final chapters he has compassionate and down-to-earth tips for families coping with terminal decisions for their loved ones and good advice on how to avoid unnecessary medicalization of the normal process of dying.

Dr. Reznik is even informative for situations in which the doctor-patient relationship has broken down. "Do not threaten the physician who is still taking care of you. This will usually just lead to an increase in defensive medicine… If you must threaten, save it for the time when this doctor is no longer caring for you or your relative. Switch to a different doctor first."

While much of the case that this book presents is discomforting, e.g., that we haven't really beat cancer, that we don't really practice "best evidence" uniformly in medicine, that vested interests of large corporate entities have directly and adversely influenced ordinary doctor-patient encounters, that we aren't going to live forever no matter what we do, and that our doctors are not omnipotent, he has adduced a sensible prescription for change. Each physician and each patient needs to change, one by one. This starts just by becoming conscious and informed in each medical decision that we make; we could have a far better health care system than we do now. This is Dr. Reznik's message.

In the end this is a very affirming book. It is affirming for physicians because it brings a lot of automatic and unconscious behaviors into focus for conscious inspection. It clearly illustrates a number of paths that can lead physicians out of the "medical box." It can have the result of relieving the average physician of the huge burden of "omnipotence." Very interesting things can happen when you don't have to be perfect anymore, where "good enough" is, well, good enough.

The bottom line he offers for patients is revolutionary—a new paradigm: "I would argue that, as in matters of personal safety, in the matters of personal health an individual has to have a choice, and no one has the right to judge this choice…When the true limits of medicine are realized and accepted, there is a possibility of more preparedness, clearer decision-making, and peace of mind. …As a physician, when I'm dealing with a patient who is comfortable refusing what I offer, I know that this person is not likely to become a victim of the system. They preserve their integrity by not putting me (and the institution of medical care) above themselves. They are more likely to live and die free."

Dr. Oleg Reznik is a very good physician. I know because I supervised his training as a family physician. He had the unusual conviction and ability to question what the "medical machine" was doing even as an intern, which created a few problems for me. In fact, this created a fair number of headaches for both of us, but that is his point. Good medicine can only occur when we acknowledge the exceptions, the unique personal circumstances and needs inherent in every situation, and deal open-mindedly with the headaches that ensue. In his training he was diligent and conscientious in support of the style of practice he aspired to, and this met my needs. This book now shows a wisdom that is very rare for a physician so early in his career. It is a brief, but accomplished synthesis of current medical data and all too common medical practices. His perspective is undeniably somewhat contrarian. To that concern I can respond, if you've been successful in all your medical encounters and have the health that you want, you probably don't need to listen to him. In all other cases it will definitely be worth your while to spend a couple of hours with this articulate and perceptive physician, accompany him as he accomplishes his rounds in the office and at the hospital, meet real patients, and share his reflections on what he has observed. In fact, I believe that you will be significantly more autonomous and healthier for it.

—Colin P Kopes-Kerr, MD, JD, MPH

Vice Chairman, Department of Family Medicine, and Program Director of the Family Medicine Residency Program, at University Hospital and SUNY Stony Brook School of Medicine, Stony Brook, NY.

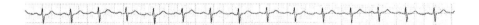

1 Introduction

Health care is becoming increasingly complex, with multiple factors affecting decision making. You may have heard about or experienced some of the shortcomings of this system first hand. People of all ages and all degrees of health are affected by the current way of medical practice. It starts with infants, who are put through a variety of tests by overzealous physicians responding to their own or their parent's fears. Young women become unnecessarily worried from their Pap smear screening, prenatal testing, and encountering a wall of defensive medicine during childbirth. Middle aged men are enticed into a highly questionable practice of prostate cancer screening and ending up with surgeries that, instead of prolonging their life, leave them deprived of their basic human capacities. There are a slew of breast biopsies and mastectomies as a result of screening mammography in women, without concomitant prolongation of life but with an enormous mental and physical toll. Finally, the elderly are put through testing and procedures in the last six months of life—the evidence now clearly shows that this actually slightly shorten their lives when compared with those who did not have the option of utilizing health care system to the same extent (due to living in regions of the US with lower Health Care funding).

When we enter the system as patients, we are simply hoping that a physician will take good care of us. We also sometimes hope that health care will prevent us from getting sick, discover and diagnose any hidden illness, cure or treat it, and possibly make us live longer. The physician of course tries to live up to some of these expectations.

I am a doctor, but this doesn't protect me from health problems. Recently, I had a kidney stone, and became a patient. The physician taking care of me in the emergency room accurately diagnosed and treated the problem. At the discharge, the physician told me that I "needed" to follow up with a urologist. Now that I have a kidney stone I should have a urologist. Those two go together in her mind. She was the usual overworked senior resident in the emergency room of a university hospital. She told me what she tells all the patients discharged after the discovery of a kidney stone. From the point of view of the usual medical training, she was an exemplary physician. She gave her recommendation with the best intentions: she truly believed that she was doing me good by giving that advice.

Physicians are systematically taught to give the same advice to everyone; we do not have the time nor the training to pay attention to individual differences.

She was quite surprised when I told her that I wasn't planning to follow her advice, that I simply intended to alter my diet. At that point I opted not to follow her medical advice and not to subject myself to additional testing with the time commitment, inconvenience, and expense that it entails, let alone the risks of false-positive results and unnecessary procedures with their side-effects. That was my personal preference. Whether or not my decisions were wise is not the issue. Rather, it is my hope to empower patients and their family members to recognize the freedom of choice even when none is presented and to know that the information they lack for decision making can be obtained by directly questioning the system. It is also my intention to decrease undue expectations that the medical system itself fosters, and to deflate the balloon of medical omnipotence.

I call this system **The Health Care Machine** because it has become mechanical. The race for 'clinical productivity' is turning health care into another form of an assembly line. There are other factors I'll soon discuss that push us in the same direction. A physician who sees you is no longer an agent who works for you. Rather, he or she is trying to balance a number of conflicting demands. As I watched a TV interview at an advertising agency that created a television ad for one of the frequently used drugs, the spokesperson stated "…the medications now are a part of a healthy lifestyle…" She truly believed that and wanted the rest of the world to believe it as well. So it is with the physicians and other health care workers who are placed in a position (and I call this position The Medical Box) that pressures them to have only a standard, mechanical response to any given set of problems. Eventually, being in that box makes them believe that those are the only possible answers. I think a patient can navigate through this system much more successfully by being aware of its limitations.

In the body of this book, I present vignettes from my clinical practice, experience in the medical school and residency, and personal research. Mostly they are the accounts of actual patients I have cared for, directly or indirectly. I have altered the details to make them unrecognizable while maintaining the essence of each story intact. They all demonstrate the facets and influences of "the rules of the game": the game of health care. It is my hope that from reading these accounts with the accompanying discussions, you will understand the motives influencing your doctor's decisions and will learn how to be more self-reliant.

Throughout the book I placed subheadings: *Patient/Family Perspective, Physician's Perspective, Societal Perspective* and *Spiritual/Philosophical Perspective.* Though these subdivisions are somewhat artificial, since to some degree, one perspective contains all of the others, I hope that they will ease the flow and absorption of the material. *Patient/Family Perspective* deals with the issues that most closely relate to, or would be most helpful for prospective patients and their families. *Physician's Perspective* reveals physicians perception of the issue. *Societal Perspective* shows the impact on the society as a whole. *Spiritual/Philosophical Perspective* addresses spiritual and philosophical aspects of medical care, aspects that cannot truly be separated from any endeavor seeking to understand a human being.

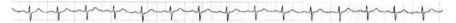

2   The Medical Box

Physician's Perspective

The term 'Medical Box' is my invention to show the boxed-in thinking imposed on physicians; the boundaries they need to overcome in order to do what's in the patient's best interest. I believe it is important for the patient to be aware of them too. Here are what I call the four corners of the Medical Box:

- Fear of litigation.
- Financial and time pressure.
- Guidelines of Health Care authorities.
- The current Medical Model—disease oriented thinking.

I think most physicians wish to do good and to be genuinely helpful. This wish is impeded by the Medical Box.

Litigation has a potential of disrupting medical practice and increasing malpractice insurance premiums. Being labeled as high risk physician limits one's employability. According to the Association of American Medical Colleges, an average physician who graduated from medical school in 2004 had $115,000 of educational debts! This debt has been steadily increasing. After spending a minimum of eleven years of intense learning, one tends to want to have some degree of comfort, to be able to repay one's debts, and have a feeling of some financial security in order to support a family. All of that is threatened by a lawsuit. Medical mistakes do happen and it is fair to hold the doctor accountable for them. However, the success of a lawsuit does not always depend on the degree or even presence of a mistake on the doctor's part, but rather, on the gravity of the outcome or on chance alone. One of my obstetrical colleagues was successfully sued after her patient's unborn baby died. Though by the standards of medical practice there was no error, it is hard for the jury not to feel overwhelmed by such a tragedy. Consequently, she was deemed guilty, resulting in stigmatization, raised malpractice insurance premium, and a mark on the record that will be questioned whenever she may want to look for another job, or apply for another malpractice insurance.

This record is permanent. It is not surprising that fear of being sued is one of the major forces driving medical decision making in the US today. I attempt to illustrate some of the implications of this in the vignettes of the subsequent chapters where actual patients are described. I am not the only one to believe that the success of a lawsuit does not depend on the presence of an error. Linda Crawford, who is on the faculty of Harvard Law School, where she teaches trial advocacy and has been consulting people on research and evidence-based effectiveness for malpractice depositions, states that five out of six lawsuits involve good medicine, half the time there isn't even a bad outcome (Tracy, 2003). She further states: "Let's talk about brain-damaged children. All of us now go into labor and delivery presuming we will have a perfect outcome. The parents believe it. The family believes it. The community believes it, and frankly the providers believe it; yet, it is still true that we have not made any significant gains since 1965. Five percent of children are born with significant disabilities. There is a gap between what everybody is expecting and the reality. I am all for good relationships with your patients; I think it has a great deal to do with the quality of our professional lives. However, I also look at the specialties and the individual surgeons who are sued, and it often has to do with the expectations of your patients going into whatever the event is." These expectations are not easily changed and are often the result of a well publicized boasting of the medical system about the great advances we've achieved.

Money and time are intimately related in our society and the medical system is no exception. Beginning in medical school, we (medical students) were repeatedly told that medicine is business. I do not share this opinion but it is now held by the vast majority of physicians. More than that, in medical school we were specifically taught that it is not important for us to care about the patients, what is important is to know how to create an impression of caring. We were then taught how to do that, how to fake a caring attitude. A doctor has to say "aha", " tell me more", to make a pause after a patient says something he finds significant; one needs to make brief remarks indicating compassion and understanding so as not to make an impression of being uncaring. All this is so that the business part of medicine can go more smoothly.

Third party payers also drive some of the important changes in this realm. Health insurance attempts to cover health care needs and make some money off of this process. They have to find some quantifiable way of reimbursing physicians. This quantification (which is difficult to avoid) is one of the problems. My residency training was in a suburban university hospital. From time to time, in addition to the usual lectures by the faculty, we were lectured by the community physicians who were supposed to teach us how to "survive in the real world". We were taught that "talking to the patient doesn't pay", that in order to survive financially we needed to decrease the amount of talk to the minimum and instead to do as many office procedures as possible. Insurance won't pay for educating a patient, but they pay for throat cultures, wart removals, hearing, vision, blood and urine tests etc. An excerpt from a recent article for the physicians in the Family Practice Management Journal (Martz, 2003) illustrates this point:

"As practices' expenses continue to grow at a faster pace than revenues, physicians are under greater pressure to do more with less. While working harder and seeing increasing numbers of patients each day is an option, finding methods to work smarter is becoming an attractive alternative. One viable strategy for your practice is to increase charges per unit of time. Performing more procedures is a simple and successful way to achieve this goal.

As you are probably aware, not all procedures are created equal. Some procedures (e.g., flexible sigmoidoscopy) are reimbursed very poorly considering the time they require. Other procedures (e.g., skin biopsy and excisions, colposcopy/biopsy and exercise treadmill testing), though reimbursed more handsomely, may require significant amounts of physician and nursing time, significant up-front costs to the practice and extensive training. However, there is another category of procedures well worth your time and effort - joint and soft-tissue injections."

I don't think that many patients want to see a physician who is thinking of performing more procedures as a means of increasing his revenue. We want our physician to be impartial keeping in mind only what's in our best interest. The interest in joint and soft tissue injections is so strong that it drives practices that were proven to have no more effect than a placebo. I still see patients who ask me to inject their knees with Synvisc—an expensive product used to treat osteoarthritis and subsequently shown to be no better than injections of salt water (Pedtgrella et al, 2002). Their previous doctor did it and insurance paid for it, so they want more. Things may soon get to the point that when you come to your doctor for a sore throat, he'll offer you a knee injection.

Another necessary way of increasing the revenue is to address one or two problems at a time and to keep bringing patient back for frequent revisits. Insurance will pay for addressing one problem on separate visits, but will question and decrease payment for trying to address multiple problems in one visit. Health insurance usually monitors physicians—this is called physician profiling. Payments are decreased to the physicians who charge more than the average. This causes a disincentive to try to solve more than one problem and a preference for younger and healthier patients with fewer problems. There is also a threat of an audit—when a health insurance such as Medicare may review charts. If during an audit, chart documentation does not reflect the charges, a practice can be fined millions of dollars. This brings several consequences. One is that physicians will 'downcode' (charge insurance less) just to avoid the possibility of an audit, another is the need for careful documentation for insurance purposes (which is not the same as the patient's); the third is less reimbursement. All three cause the physician to accelerate his pace in order to continue making the same amount of money. Naturally, quality suffers. Dealing with insurance leads to an additional loss of time because of other bureaucratic processes involved. Billing, coding, credentialing, and auditing are the tasks that take the time and money. For example, a physician has to hire a biller or a billing service. Different insurance companies use different drug formularies—list of medications that are preferentially covered. The physician has to be able to keep up with all that and have the time to do quite a bit for the patient—what the guidelines demand, and what the patient wants, which are usually two different things.

Most medications and treatments carry some consequences, as does the option of foregoing them. That and the fact that physicians have been required to have the informed consent of a patient, creates tension. On the one hand, the physician has to educate the patient in order to obtain a true informed consent; on the other hand, he has no time/money for doing that, but if something adverse should happen a physician can be successfully sued by the patient if there was no written or verbal informed consent.

I would like to digress a bit to discuss informed consent. Informed consent was created with an intention to help the patient make an independent decision about their health care, to actively participate in their health care and be protected from authoritarian physicians. With time, and under the above mentioned pressures, it has degenerated. Informed consent seems mainly to be the tool to protect the doctor, not the patient, and it can do harm. A physician now obtains informed consent because this protects him from being sued. If an adverse outcome occurs, a doctor says—"we discussed this and the patient consented," thus the doctor is off the hook. There is usually no true education taking place, and often the risks are presented only after the patient was already thoroughly convinced by the doctor and made up his mind to do what the doctor wants him to do. I will discuss why a doctor may *want* you to do something below. The other harm of an informed consent is a nocebo effect (O'Mathúna, 2003). It is the opposite of the placebo effect, which is a beneficial effect of a neutral substance after a suggestion that it can do good. A nocebo effect is an adverse effect of a neutral substance or treatment after a suggestion that it can do harm. Research has found effects such as drowsiness, headache, fatigue, sensation of heaviness, and nausea after patients took a neutral substance with a suggestion that it is a medication that can cause side-effects.

Now back to why the physician may *want* you to do one thing or another, to take medications, to undergo tests and procedures. The obvious response is that they are concerned about your health and want you to be well and live longer. This indeed is frequently the case. Other pressures however will often cloud these good intentions and even the physician himself may not be aware of some of his own motives. **Guidelines of healthcare authorities** (i.e. American College of Cardiology, The United States Preventive Services Task Force) are designed to help the doctor practice the best up to date medicine. Qualified physicians review the available scientific evidence and come up with the best treatment options for each disease. When there is a lack of evidence, a "consensus expert opinion" is formed.

In an ideal situation, a physician's role would be to discuss these treatment recommendations with the patient and form a plan according to the patient's individual differences and personal preferences. In actuality, as we discussed above, there is a lack of time for providing true education for a patient. But, more importantly, there is a fear of litigation. "What will I say in court," thinks a physician, "when this patient or his family sues me after a heart attack." How will I explain why I did not have him on this drug, the drug that is recommended by the health care authorities. Therefore a physician feels uncomfortable with a patient who does not follow all "expert recommendations", usually labeling such patient as non-compliant, a term that helps to get off the hook later in court. It is far more comfortable for a general practitioner to send a patient for multiple studies and to multiple specialists then trying to shoulder the responsibility alone. This leads to many unnecessary consultations and tests, some of which, as we shall see later, bring harm. And, as we shall see, the specialists then have their own pressures.

Finally, **the current medical model,** as discussed in the article *The End of the Disease Era* (Tinetti, 2004), presents a challenge. It is a model based on treating acute conditions that is now applied to all of medicine. In this model, we look for a pattern of symptoms and findings that fit the definition of a certain disease. We than label the person—"you have disease X, here is the algorithm for its treatment." The problem arises when a person does not clearly fit into a particular label. As we became a longer living society we have accumulated more and more people who fall into the category of this poorly defined illness. A physician usually feels very uncomfortable treating the symptom that he cannot label as a specific illness. The physician's discomfort at least in part has to do with a legal fear. If an adverse reaction occurs to a medication that he is prescribing without its indicated use (each medication is indicated and usually FDA approved for treating certain diseases), he may be in trouble. How will he justify the reasons for using it? Medical education also teaches physicians not to focus on treating the symptoms but to treat an underlying disease. For the patient, on the other hand, it is the symptom that matters most. This, as mentioned in the article, leads to undertreatment, overtreatment, and mistreatment. It will be discussed in more detail in the chapter dedicated to this topic—The Medical Model.

Another aspect of the disease model is the use of various screening and preventive measures that physicians are asked to do by the makers of guidelines. This then places them into an impossible position. The United States Preventive Services Task Force, which is one of the major agencies recommending preventive medical services in the US, found approximately fifty preventive services to be effective (Coffield, 2001). Examples are: providing tobacco cessation counseling to adults, counseling adolescents on drug and alcohol abstinence, screening adults for colorectal cancer, screening young women for chlamydial infection, screening adults for problem drinking and domestic violence, vaccination, visual impairment in adults over sixty five years of age...the list goes on and on. In fact it has been estimated that, on average, adult patients have approximately a dozen risk factors requiring approximately twenty four preventive services (Coffield, 2001). A primary care physician is required to provide these services or face the risk of being blamed and held responsible for not providing them. One of the ways of getting out of this predicament for a physician is to document that the patient who resisted having all of the required procedures and tests is non-compliant, or to get rid of the patient altogether by discharging him from the practice. Genuinely discussing patients' priorities with the patient, obtaining a true informed consent and documenting it (for possible future legal defense) is a luxury that few physicians can afford.

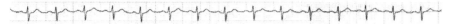

3   The Case of a Man with Chest Pains

Patient/Family Perspective

This was a patient who came to the resident clinic and was seen by one of my senior residents. In residency, after seeing each patient, a resident precepts with an attending physician who supervises and teaches. The resident then goes back to the patient with final recommendations. This was an eighty-six year old man who came to the clinic out of his wife's insistence. His wife had wanted him to see a doctor for a few years at that stage, because of occasional chest discomfort. He was a retired owner of a landscaping company. During his retirement he attended to their garden, did some rebuilding of their house, and walked to the beach a couple of times per week during the summer to do some fishing. Their house was about a mile and a half away from the beach. From time to time he would get chest tightness while waking fast or going up the stairs. This never lasted more than a few minutes and always went away as soon as he stopped and rested. He'd been having these pains over the previous couple of years, but tried to avoid seeing a doctor and took no medications. The symptoms hadn't changed since he started having them few years back, he did not consider them too bothersome and was generally satisfied with his current state of health. His physical examination and office ECG were unremarkable.

Physician's Perspective

As I heard this resident present the case I recognized, as did the other resident, that this was a case of what we call a chronic stable angina. It is a chronic chest pain usually related to blockages in the arteries supplying the heart muscle. It is quite reasonable to offer a trial of medical management—prescribe a few pills, in a case like this (ACC/AHA 2002 guideline update) and see if symptoms will improve. The range of possible interventions could be from doing nothing (if the patient prefers it that way in spite of a medical recommendation to take a medication) to performing some non-invasive tests such as a stress test (walking on a treadmill or getting an injection of a medication and monitoring the heart) and echocardiogram (ultrasound of the heart), if the patient wanted to go in the direction of aggressive early intervention. Sending a patient to a cardiologist is reasonable too, but arranging for a coronary angiography as the first procedure is an overkill. Coronary angiography is an invasive procedure in which a catheter is introduced into a large artery in the groin and threaded up into the heart to look at its blood vessels—coronary arteries. It is an overkill, because it's an invasive procedure with side-effects. Such a procedure is warranted when there is an indication that the patient is at risk, and that risk outweighs the risk of a procedure. "Primum Non Nocere" ("at first, do no harm") is a maxim from the Hippocratic oath taken by most physicians.

Non-invasive tests are usually done first, to determine whether the risk of an invasive procedure would be justified. When a non-invasive procedure is negative—the patient is not likely to benefit from the invasive one, while the risks remain. The patient and the physician have to be aware that by accepting a coronary angiography, one gets on the conveyor belt that can lead to other procedures such as angioplasty with placement of stents, or coronary artery bypass surgery. Angioplasty is a procedure whereby a small balloon is inflated inside the blood vessel that has a narrowing thus stretching it back open. A stent, which is a metal spring-like structure, is then placed to prevent the re-expanded blood vessel from closing right back. Coronary artery bypass graft surgery is as major a surgery as one could think of. The chest is sawed open and grafts (either a small artery from the chest or veins from the leg, or both) are used to connect the big artery (aorta) with the heart arteries that are compromised by a narrowing. To do that, the heart sometimes has to be temporarily stopped.

The resident intentionally did not discuss options with the patient, knowing that this was a loaded issue. A patient with a complaint of chest pain, no matter how innocuous, could end up having a heart attack, as can anyone who does not have a chest pain for that matter. But in this case, the doctor can be blamed for not preventing it. The resident accurately enumerated the patient's options. The supervising physician promptly replied—"when this patient has a heart attack and you are in court, what will you say then?" The resident went along with the idea of defensive medicine and proposed to send this patient to arrange for a coronary angiography. For that she called a cardiologist with whom she'd done a rotation earlier and whom she liked. The resident then went back to the patient with the goal of convincing him to do the "right thing." If the patient would have declined her proposal, she would label him as non-compliant to provide herself with some degree of comfort.

Patient/Family Perspective

This old man didn't want to defy his new doctor and went along. He essentially made up his mind without hearing about the possible side-effects of the procedure, including heart attack, stroke, cardiac arrhythmias, cardiac tamponade (bleeding into the sac that surrounds the heart that leads to rapid heart failure), trauma to the artery caused by hematoma (bleeding around the groin artery), hemorrhage, reaction to contrast medium (a dye injected to visualize blood vessels on X-ray) and others. Generally, the risk of serious complications ranges from 1 in 1,000 to 1 in 500 (MedlinePlus). Coronary artery bypass graft surgery has more dangers, including, among others 1 to 2 % risk of death, risks of kidney failure, stroke, decline in memory and other cognitive functions (Knipp et al, 2004; Hunt et al, 2000; Ho et al, 2004; Mayo Clinic 2004). Successful surgeries are well publicized, such as ones of David Letterman and President Clinton, but people who wake up after a surgery with brain damage usually remain known only to their families.

Even a benign-appearing non-invasive test such as a cardiac exercise stress test, for example, has side-effects. Among patients undergoing this test, eight in 10,000 will have some serious complication such as a heart attack, serious arrhythmia, or death; death specifically occurs in one in 20,000 (Ellestad, 1980).

In the case of our patient, I think it is important to point out that the decision was made without giving the patient the benefit of education and choice. Subsequently, an "informed consent" would be obtained to insure that physician was protected in case something went wrong during the procedure. The dialog I reported between the resident and supervisor is akin to the inner dialog that goes on in the minds of many physicians.

A few weeks later, I heard about this patient again. He underwent coronary angiography and some blockages were found. It is not at all surprising that an eighty six year old person would have some blockages in the coronary arteries, regardless of whether they have any chest pains or not. What made this case stick in my memory was that not only was the first angiography in my opinion unnecessary but now he was going for a second one. This was because the cardiologist to whom he was originally sent could perform only diagnostic procedures because of the kind of facility he worked at (his hospital did not have a backup of a cardiothoracic surgeon). To actually fix the problem, this old man now had to go to another cardiologist who had to repeat angiography and fix the plumbing—

blockage in one of the blood vessels of the heart. This "fixing" however was not of any proven benefit. Medical scientific evidence shows that opening blood vessels works in an acute heart attack, and in unstable (worsening) angina, but not in chronic stable angina in an 86 year old patient.

Physician's Perspective

The New York Times magazine presented an interview of two top heart experts by Gina Kolata in March 21, 2004 (Kolata, 2004, excerpted with permission from the New York Times magazine). They were Dr. David Brown, an interventional cardiologist at Beth Israel Medical Center in New York and Dr. David Waters, a cardiologist at the University of California at San Francisco. The reporter says, "...the old idea was this: Coronary disease is akin to sludge building up in a pipe. Plaque accumulates slowly, over decades, and once it is there it is pretty much there for good. Every year, the narrowing grows more severe until one day no blood can get through and the patient has a heart attack. Bypass surgery or angioplasty — opening arteries by pushing plaque back with a tiny balloon and then, often, holding it there with a stent — can open up a narrowed artery before it closes completely. And so, it was assumed, heart attacks could be averted.

But, researchers say, *most heart attacks do not occur because an artery is narrowed by plaque. Instead, they say, heart attacks occur when an area of plaque bursts, a clot forms over the area and blood flow is abruptly blocked. In 75 to 80 percent of cases, the plaque that erupts was not obstructing an artery and would not be stented or bypassed. The dangerous plaque is soft and fragile, produces no symptoms and would not be seen as an obstruction to blood flow.*" (my emphasis)

"[…] Instead, recent and continuing studies show that a more powerful way to prevent heart attacks in patients at high risk is to adhere rigorously to what can seem like boring old advice — giving up smoking, for example, and taking drugs to get blood pressure under control, drive cholesterol levels down and prevent blood clotting."

Since this was not my patient, I did not hear about him again but do hope that no harm came to him. The physicians were made to feel better by reassuring themselves that they did "all that could be done" and safer by knowing that after all the procedures, even if the patient died of a heart attack, no one could blame them since they carried out the standard recommendations, and involved a specialist to give this patient every possible "advantage."

Here I would like to speak of some of the reasons that the specialists agree to give these kinds of "advantages." A succinct answer comes again from the New York Times article mentioned above (Kolata, 2004) "… Dr. David Hillis, an interventional cardiologist at the University of Texas Southwestern Medical Center in Dallas, explained: 'If you're an invasive cardiologist and Joe Smith, the local internist, is sending you patients, and if you tell them they don't need the procedure, pretty soon Joe Smith doesn't send patients anymore. Sometimes you can talk yourself into doing it even though in your heart of hearts you don't think it's right.'

"Dr. Topol said a patient typically goes to a cardiologist with a vague complaint like indigestion or shortness of breath, or because a scan of the heart indicated calcium deposits — a sign of atherosclerosis, or buildup of plaque. The cardiologist puts the patient in the cardiac catheterization room, examining the arteries with an angiogram. Since most people who are middle-aged and older have atherosclerosis, the angiogram will more often than not show a narrowing. Inevitably, the patient gets a stent."

"'It's this train where you can't get off at any station along the way,' Dr. Topol said. 'Once you get on the train, you're getting the stents. Once you get in the cath lab, it's pretty likely that something will get done.'"

"Even more disquieting,' Dr. Topol said, 'is that stenting can actually cause minor heart attacks in about four percent of patients. That can add up to a lot of people suffering heart damage from a procedure meant to prevent it."

"'It has not been a welcome thought,' Dr. Topol said."

Patient/Family Perspective

Now what of our patient, what would I want him to have done if he was my loved one, a family member or a friend? I think that first he needs to start with an attitude that a doctor is someone who can provide information and opinion but not someone to rely upon in making decisions. One can see a physician like a painter whom one hires to paint one's house. A painter can give his expert opinions and advice but cannot make the final decision. Why not? Because he does not know who you are as a human being, what is important to him may not be important to you. And if you really want to paint your bedroom purple, you'll do it even if your painter finds it distasteful. We need not discount our nature and what is important to us in life and relegate decision making to a physician. We know ourselves better than anyone else can know us.

He should have approached this as any other decision in his life, asked what options there were. If not satisfied with the options given to him, he could have asked for more options. He needed to know about the risks and benefits of doing the procedures, of taking medicines alone, or of doing nothing at all. He should have asked about the accuracy of the test. In my opinion, when nothing seems like a good option, it is better to do nothing than to rush in. Asking for another opinion and looking for other alternatives may be appropriate. No doubt he would have encountered some resistance from his doctor because of the numerous reasons discussed above. But he would be able to make a better decision for himself.

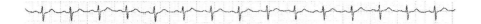

4 The Case of Threatening the Doctor

Patient/Family Perspective

This was a fifty-eight year old man who'd suffered a major stroke a year prior to his admission to the hospital. The stroke had paralyzed the right side of his body, he could speak only a few words mainly saying yes or no, and suffered from seizures. He lived at a nursing home and was brought to the hospital because of fever and cough. I was a senior resident on the team that took care of him during this admission to the hospital. In spite of the significant neurological deficits, as far as we could tell he understood everything that went on. His family confirmed that his mind was clear. He was not what one can call a difficult patient. People who took care of him found him pleasant and friendly. We felt genuine compassion for this man who was not old but had suffered a great deal.

Both the medical team and the patient's family knew what was going on: another aspiration pneumonia. Patients, after a significant stroke and those who have seizures, are predisposed to getting them. When the muscles of the throat do not function properly, swallowing is disrupted and some of the food content is inhaled, ending up in the lungs and sometimes causing a pneumonia. He had been admitted to the hospital a few weeks prior for the same thing. At that time he was taken care of by another team of doctors. He continued to have seizures as well. From the record of a prior admission, we saw that adequate seizure control could not be achieved because of the side effects of the medications. The type of seizures this patient suffered was not likely to cause aspiration. It was not known whether swallowing difficulty, seizure, poor breathing pattern, or a combination of factors caused patient's pneumonia. The family was quite angry, they felt that the medical system has failed them and they tried to get a better level of care by threats and intimidation. They approached our attending (supervising) physician and stated that they had a relative at the department of health and unless their loved one was now better taken care of, they would report and investigate the physicians managing him.

Physician's Perspective

In our age of litigation this produced an immediate outcome, though probably not the one that family truly desired. Our attending physician became genuinely frightened. He then responded with the usual strategy used in these situations. He demonstrated an outward agreement with the family and stated that "everything" would be done and done immediately. This pacified the family for a short while. The ensuing events were not in the patient's best interest, but provided proof to potential investigators that everything possible was being done. When a patient is not doing well and there is a risk of a lawsuit, a physician will often go into this mode. In a situation like that, it does not matter so much whether or not the patient improves. What becomes important is that all of the guidelines have been followed, all possible therapies tried, all possible consultants consulted. In this process the patient usually suffers from the unnecessary procedures and tests and often undergoes futile treatments just to prove to possible future investigators that the doctor cannot be blamed.

Patient/Family Perspective

A CT scan and an MRI of the brain were done for our patient, followed by CT scan of the chest and abdomen. Neurology was consulted to evaluate the patient regarding his seizures and a possibility of another stroke, and to improve seizure control. A Gastroenterology consultant was called in to place a gastric tube, and after several unsuccessful attempts (it can be a technically challenging procedure), general surgery was consulted and did succeed in placing a gastric tube after all. Initially, it was thought that these tubes could decrease incidents of aspiration pneumonia. In reality, the data on these tubes (also called PEG—percutaneous endoscopic gastrostomy tube) say that they are rarely effective in doing so. They will not increase comfort; they will not prolong life, and they are associated with their own adverse effects (Katsura et al, 1898; Bath et al. 1999). With regard to these tubes, the initial thinking was that since a patient does not need to swallow he is protected against an aspiration. This did not turn out to be the case in the elderly and sick patients. They continued to aspirate after regurgitating food. The tube itself can become problematic when the opening in the abdominal wall gets infected. But a team of doctors motivated by an insistent family, who also threatened them, were willing to do almost anything to show that "everything" was being done. To perform all of these procedures, the patient required multiple daily blood tests to monitor drug levels and side effects, multiple X-rays, and prolonged periods of time without food. Finally, after a week's stay, patient was discharged on more medication and with a stomach tube.

Three days later, the patient was back with fever again. The family were beside themselves. The patient smiled when the admitting resident gently said to him "So John, you really like us, you are back." He seemed resigned to his physical condition, but not depressed. We were impressed at the ease with which he accepted his suffering. The family demanded to speak to the doctor who was in charge of the department. At that point our residency program director was summoned. He was a man of uncommon courage and compassion. He also held a law degree in addition to the medical degree. He explained to the family that the patient's condition was such that he was bound to have recurrent problems and no amount of medical care could make him well, that this was likely to continue until he would pass away. What we could do was to try to manage these problems as they came up, try to decrease his discomfort. The family was astounded to hear that, but were able to accept it and changed their attitude drastically. They did not blame as much and did not demand more procedures. This patient was shortly discharged and returned much less frequently, as the family accepted less aggressive management. More treatments were done at the nursing home where the patient lived.

In reflecting upon this case, I would not recommend to patients and their families that they threaten physicians while they are still in their care. An attempt at an honest and open discussion in a non-threatening atmosphere would yield better results. If you are not happy with the treatment you get, ask for a second opinion or switch care altogether to another physician by speaking to a patient representative at the hospital.

A non-medical person threatening a medical system can be compared to a blind person wandering onto the highway and threatening the upcoming ten-wheeler trucks. Whether or not there was a malpractice, if your loved one is still being treated, it is not a good time to go to war since your loved one may become one of the casualties. The courage of the physician who was willing to speak openly to the family is uncommon. Most physicians are afraid that this openness will be taken as resignation or giving up that will anger the family. This does happen sometimes.

There is another aspect here that is worth mentioning and that I will discuss in more detail in the chapter—*The Case of Unreasonable Expectations, Family Guilt and Blame*. It has been my experience on multiple occasions that the family that feels guilty about putting the patient into a nursing home rather than caring for him or her at home, tend to be excessively fervent in demanding excellent care from others (the hospital and nursing home personnel). These may be the ways of relieving their guilt feelings by attempting to prove to themselves that they really care. I would recommend anyone for whom this may be true to shed all guilt (by psychotherapy or other means) before becoming involved with the care of a loved one. You have done what you could, and stories about what "a good child should be doing for his parents" is just a standard that someone, no matter how authoritative, came up with. It does not need to be followed and should not make you feel bad. This facilitates better decision making, more love and less blame.

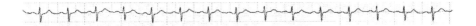

5 The Case of a Sinking Ship

Patient/Family Perspective

This was a forty-seven year old man with AIDS who was admitted to the hospital because of fever and cough. X-ray findings were inconclusive and showed a possible mild pneumonia. He was treated with the usual: antibiotics, intravenous fluid and oxygen. His fever and cough resolved, but he continued to feel sick. Particularly, he now complained more of abdominal pain and nausea. After some additional blood tests, we discovered that he suffered from an acute pancreatitis, a very dangerous condition, particularly in a debilitated patient. Fever and cough on his initial presentation could have been a "red herring" caused by an upper respiratory illness, they could have been caused by the pancreatitis that was missed, pancreatitis could have been precipitated by the acute illness, by the interaction of the HIV medication with the antibiotics we were giving, or could have been there coincidentally as a result of any number of causes. It was really impossible to know. We did the appropriate investigations, restricted his diet, stopped the possibly offending medications and waited, but his respiratory status started to deteriorate. The patient was appreciative of the care he received and we shared all information with him openly. The medical system had helped him on multiple occasions in the past. His former wife visited him but did not participate in medical decision-making. He understood the seriousness of his condition.

Physician's Perspective

At that time we (the residents) were supervised by one of the senior faculty members. After discussing the case we suspected that the patient was experiencing one of the known and very lethal complications—ARDS (acute respiratory distress syndrome). Our supervising physician then told us to obtain pulmonary, gastroenterology, and infectious disease consultations. The pulmonary consultation was necessary since there was a high probability of this patient needing a transfer to the intensive care unit, getting intubated, and needing mechanical ventilation (a machine that will breathe for him). We questioned why other consultations were needed. With a look of a wise man, and after a short pause, our teaching physician said, "when your ship is sinking, bring everyone down with you." The patient had all of the consultations. As a result of the consultants' recommendations he had blood and urine cultures, some further slight changes of medications, a few additional blood tests. He passed away a few days later in the intensive care unit, while on the ventilator, from multiorgan system failure. As residents we always wondered (and I still do) whether we did something wrong or didn't do enough. Sometimes it was apparent what could have been done better or differently, but almost never was it possible to make a cause and effect relationship and we would have to learn to accept this uncertainty and move on trying to do our best with the next patient.

The problem of a "sinking ship" is pervasive in medicine and touches not only patients who are not doing well but almost every patient. In other words, even if the ship is not sinking, the physician is tempted to 'bring more people on board', just in case it sinks in the future. This way personal responsibility can be diffused or eliminated by transferring it to others. The result is many trivial consultations and further fragmentation of patient care. At best, such "care" brings nothing to the patient, but usually the patient suffers further discomfort and pain without additional benefit. The specialists are well aware of this game and can hardly be blamed for proceeding with their armamentarium after a generalist asks for them. Naturally, there are also many instances when the generalist truly needs to seek the help of a specialist, and when a specialist provides a truly valuable input.

When a specialist is called for what I call 'a defensive consultation,' he will do what is necessary to cover himself. This usually requires tests. The patient either has to go through the tests or refuse them. The doctor is protected in either case. If all the tests are done, then "everything" was done. If the patient refused, then it's the fault of the patient. In either case the doctor is protected. The specialists are sometimes secretly hoping that the patient will refuse the procedure knowing that it is not necessary, but are afraid to state this openly, because that exposes them to risk. They may sometimes have a vested interest in performing certain tests or procedures. This on one occasion was the case with a gastroenterology fellow (a doctor who is in training to become a gastroenterologist) who needed to have more endoscopies. Training in any field of medicine requires a certain number of procedures done, patients seen, etc. Until he completed his numbers, we were able to get an endoscopy on anyone we requested. We could obtain it for any reason, whether it was truly indicated, or needed for the doctor's or the patient's false sense of reassurance, and for defensive purposes.

Patient/Family Perspective

The AIDS sufferer of this example was too sick to make decisions about his care in the last days of his life. He trusted the system and the system did take care of him for the most part, but also caused some unnecessary pain. If this was my loved one, I would ask the doctors who want to call for a consultation what they hope to gain from each consultant. It is poor care to call a consultant without notifying the patient or a family member. In this example the doctors would say the infectious disease consultant will help manage HIV medications and make sure that no other infectious process is going on since the patient had fever on admission. Doctors would say that a pulmonologist is needed because a patient's breathing is getting worse and the pulmonologist would be the person to manage mechanical ventilation. The gastroenterologist might be able to identify causes for the problem that were not seen since the pancreas falls into his area of specialization. When the specialist shows up and completes his evaluation, ask him *what will be his recommendations*. If he says "some tests", don't let him off the hook but inquire about three things. First, *what he is trying to find out by testing*. Second, *how this additional information is going to affect medical management* and prognosis. Third, *what testing entails*, for example, how many blood tests, what are the risks of testing (CT scan contrast can cause kidney failure, angiography can cause a stroke), does the patient have to be kept without food for long periods of time. With this information, one can decide whether additional testing is worth while.

Do not panic and assume that if you let the doctors do everything they want, the best will be done. That is not necessarily true in our age of defensive medicine. If a specialist recommends changes in management such as changing the doses of medications, adding new medications, undergoing procedures or surgery, ask how much improvement is it likely to produce and what are the chances of adverse effects. I would recommend to ask this in an open and friendly fashion, not to frighten the doctor and cause more defensiveness. As I described in the previous chapters, physicians feel a great deal of threat from litigation. One of the signs of a better doctor is one who gives you true choices about your medical management. A good physician will not impose any measure that can cause harm, even a small chance of harm.

In this case, consultations resulted in some extra blood tests to quench the physician's fear. In the next chapter I will discuss a case of a patient getting a number of unnecessary tests because of a combination of the family's indecision and the physician's position of defensiveness.

6 The Case of Death in the Emergency Room

Patient/Family Perspective

This was a patient of mine shortly after I completed my residency training and joined a practice. She was a sweet, demented, Spanish speaking ninety-two year old lady with a number of medical problems, including congestive heart failure, diabetes, high blood pressure, and insufficiency of kidney function. She lived with her daughter who brought her to the office from time to time. She did not have health insurance. I enjoyed interacting with this family, they were appreciative of the care they received. Even though they paid out of pocket, they did not have excessively high demands. The visits would involve adjustment of medications and periodic blood tests required when one takes certain medicines. We would discuss and test very selectively to decrease the cost and at the same time not to increase risks too much.

Physician's Perspective

The daughter called me one Friday evening when our clinic was closing, with the information that her mother seemed to have abdominal pain and appeared quite sick. I recognized that this matter needed special attention, and sat down to have a talk. I did not know what was going on with her mother. I proposed to her to consider the situation with a certain perspective and to discuss it with her family. One option would be to take her mother (the patient) to ER where investigative tests would be done and treatments attempted. Considering her mother's age and other medical problems, it is less likely that medical interventions would be helpful in any serious condition, no matter what this problem is. One cannot know in advance how helpful a medical intervention would be. Bringing the patient to ER would always result in some diagnostic testing, which involves some degree of suffering, but could also provide medications to relieve suffering. The family was also aware of the cost of the ER visit.

The second, in my opinion equally reasonable option, was to keep the patient home and try to provide comfort measures, such as offering water and pain relief. If the daughter accepted this option, she had to be aware of the possibility of her mother passing away at home and needed to be mentally prepared for it. I recommended that she should discuss this with other family members and come to a decision.

Patient/Family Perspective

They did not call the doctor on call that weekend. The following week I learned of what happened from the report of an ER physician. Apparently the patient was brought to the hospital on the following night. After getting a number of blood tests, electrocardiogram, and CT scan, she passed away in the ER. Resuscitation was not attempted per the family's wishes. Based on the tests the diagnosis was acute cholecystitis, which is an inflammation of the gallbladder as a result of obstructing gallstones or for other reasons.

I wrote a letter to the family expressing my condolences. I did not speak of it, but regretted that she passed away after being tested on. I could not blame them, since life and death decisions about the family members are probably the hardest decisions to make. I wandered if I was at fault. It is still not possible to know which of the two options I proposed would have been better or if another better option existed.

Physician's Perspective

The area of end of life care is challenging to both patients and doctors. As doctors we are taught that we are supposed to bring it up in our discussion with the patient, but we do not have the time, and it makes us uncomfortable. Rather than addressing this topic in haste, most physicians opt not to address it at all. The patient and his family are the only people who could take this responsibility. It will rarely get adequate attention in the Emergency Room. An ER physician will do the tests first in order to try to find the diagnosis. No one will ask the family whether their elderly and debilitated relative should or should not receive any treatment. The ER doctor reasonably assumes that, since the patient was brought to ER, investigation and treatment are desired, at least initially. It is for situations like this that many nursing homes will offer besides the 'Do Not Resuscitate' and 'Do Not Intubate' options, a 'Do Not Hospitalize' option (and sometimes other restrictions such as 'No Intravenous Fluids' and 'No Antibiotics'). This allows a selected patient to pass away with more dignity. Hospitalization, with its testing and interventions, while often life-saving, can also be dehumanizing. As hospital patients, we are considered as subjects to be tested and manipulated, hopefully to help us. As the chances of improvement and reasons for aggressive actions diminish, which is the case in a sick, very elderly, and demented patient, we are more likely to be dehumanized and less likely to be helped. Guilty feelings, such as— "perhaps we should have done more earlier so we'll do more now to compensate," also bring more damage.

Patient/Family Perspective

If this patient was my family member, I hope that I would have the strength to shed guilt and fear and act out of love only. It is not possible to give instructions on what to do in every possible case, but one can usually figure out in the moment what is the right thing to do. If you decide not to involve major medical establishments, you have to be prepared to handle death on your own. For that, one has to be able to face one's own mortality without fear. A physician or a hospice program (inpatient or outpatient) can help with comfort measures. If you decide to have everything done—tell that to the doctors, they will often assume so anyway. If you want evaluation to make a diagnosis and give you the prognosis, you have to be aware of the limitation of the medical system. First, diagnostic tests and procedures often involve discomfort, inconvenience, or pain, and can sometimes lead one in a wrong direction by giving false-positive results. Second, sometimes diagnosis can not be firmly established even with the best of tests, procedures, and consultations. Third, even if the diagnosis is established, it doesn't yield accurate predictions of what will happen in the future nor the time scale for changes. Thus if you decide to pursue this direction, you have to be prepared to stop and not to get caught into the 'Ulysses Syndrome' (see more on that in the chapter entitled *Ulysses Syndrome and the Case of an Endless Search for Reassurance*.)

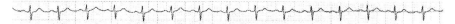

7 The Case of C-section for Breech

Physician's Perspective

One afternoon in the office I was paged by the nurses at the Labor and Delivery department and told that one of my patients presented in early labor and that the baby's position was breech. This was a twenty-eight year old Spanish-speaking lady pregnant with her second baby at 38 weeks gestation (due in two weeks). I saw her regularly for prenatal care, and as most women, she hoped to have a normal vaginal birth.

When I was told that the position was breech (bottom down instead of head down), I did what I was supposed to do—call and consult the obstetrician on call to come for a cesarean delivery. I was on my way to assist. As usual, thoughts were running through my mind questioning whether I did all that I could have done. The available data seems to say that perinatal morbidity and mortality (the chances of the baby having injury or death during the process of birthing) increases in babies born vaginally in breech position. The risk is one in a hundred, versus one in a thousand if the baby is delivered by a cesarean section (Gifford et al, 1995). Most of this difference is due to injury (0.89%) not death (0.21%), with a total increase in the combined outcome of injury or death of 1.1%. This is the best current data, though its accuracy has been questioned. Recently this has been translated into a recommendation not to deliver breach vaginally. If breech position is detected on a prenatal visit at 38 weeks, we would arrange for an option of what is called an 'external cephalic version' or schedule a cesarean delivery at 39 week's gestation. In external cephalic version, two physicians try to turn the baby's head down by applying significant manual force to certain points of the mother's abdomen. The baby is continuously monitored, and if there are signs of distress, an emergency cesarean delivery is performed.

Breech is infrequent, occurring in 3-4% of labors. Most of breech position babies detected earlier in pregnancy will turn at the end of pregnancy (Gabbe: Obstetrics - Normal and Problem Pregnancies, 4th ed., 2002).

I wondered why I had not detected it earlier in the course of prenatal care, perhaps it would have been detected by a more experienced obstetrician. This may or may not be so, but the end result would not have been very different, the patient would still be headed either for cesarean delivery or an attempt at version which is successful only half the time and has its own risks.

Patient/Family Perspective

I spoke briefly with the patient. She was somewhat disappointed at the need for C-section but trusted that this was the best. The obstetrician had already gone over the reasons for the procedure and obtained an "informed consent" which is required prior to all surgical procedures. He was one of the "old timers", and one of my favorite obstetricians.

Physician's Perspective

I generally enjoy working with the older doctors, those who are now in their sixties and more. They have lived and practiced in an era when medicine was quite different. Talking to them, I can feel and imagine how it was and almost cherish this warm memory of the past, when medicine was a lot less litigious and less business-like. In those days a doctor felt freer to consider what was better for the patients. The old timers are also less likely to blame and accuse when a patient is not doing well. Some of them, however, became disappointed and morose in response to the changes of time. So when troubles come, the old timers are generally better to be around than the docs of the past twenty years.

As I was scrubbing in to assist in the C-section, I asked him when was the last time that he delivered breech vaginally. He responded with a subtle tone of regret in his voice that it had been three to four years now. He said, in the past we gave options to the woman, telling her about the possible risks and letting her decide. Some would want to proceed with a vaginal delivery and others would opt for a cesarean. Now we simply tell them that it's unsafe for the baby to be delivered vaginally, and everyone goes for a cesarean.

Patient/Family Perspective

This example precisely illustrates how current informed consent is an illusion. The same information can be presented in a completely different way by making some subtle changes in how it is presented. The patient then has an illusion of having an option and agreeing or disagreeing with it. It is not easy for the patient to obtain objective information, especially when a decision needs to be made quickly.

Physician's Perspective

I did not blame the old timer. I could not expect him to be a hero and expose himself to risks. In fact, as I mentioned earlier, he is one of my favorite colleagues. Simply by being friendly and readily available for help, he improves the quality of care of my patients and my quality of life. The patient's position here again is not easy. While for now it seems true that the risks to the baby are lower if it is delivered by cesarean, this truth may not be absolute and may not last very long.

Societal Perspective

Rates of C-sections are rising in the US and everywhere in the world. At the present time, about one in four women delivering in the US will have a cesarean delivery. This increase is happening, in my opinion, mainly as a result of multiple lawsuits and under the pretext of improving care. For example, women who had a C-section once cannot have a vaginal birth in most places in the US because of an increased risk of complications. This policy was based on studies that were not of highest quality but did show a risk of uterine rupture of 0.2 to 9 percent depending on the type of previous incision. The risk of the baby dying was 0.13% with vaginal delivery after C-section and 0.01% if you went straight for C-section the second time without trying to give birth vaginally (Odibo et al, 2003). According to these data, the risk is very small, but still it is ten times higher than if we go straight to C-section. But this equation is not so simple. Women who undergo C-sections are more likely to have blood transfusions, infections, and as was discovered more recently, a two fold increased risk (0.05% versus 0.1%) of unexplained stillbirth (baby dying late in pregnancy before the woman goes into labor) in subsequent pregnancies (Smith et al, 2004). This study is likely to be ignored for a while, because the consequence is not immediate and the cause and effect relationship cannot be fully established; hence it is not likely to result in a successful lawsuit. As we will see in the following chapter, physicians are actually encouraged (behind closed doors) to increase the rate of C-sections because it decreases the losses due to lawsuits. As long as the immediate result seems better the physicians will continue to be encouraged by the malpractice insurance companies to perform more C-sections.

Patient/Family Perspective

If this patient was my loved one, I would hope that she would not accept the information given by a physician without questioning, especially if she wanted to have a vaginal birth. I hope that she would trust her own feelings and her intuition and when not satisfied with the physician's proposal would question it. Specifically what are the actual risks? How good is the quality of the data that this information is based upon? Are there studies or authorities questioning the accuracy of the data? Look for the data yourself. As we know in medicine, we'll usually offer major surgery with a mortality risk of 1% without thinking twice. Why is it then that here we are so bothered by the risk that is a lot smaller? Few physicians read the data critically. Most simply follow the recommendations handed down by the authorities. These authorities are often helpful in sorting out the data but are not exempt from error and bias. It is a lot safer for a physician to simply follow the guidelines. The next question should be—"Are there other doctors who would do things your way?" If so, and such doctors and midwives do exist, ask to speak to them as a second opinion. If they are not available at the hospital where you are, inquire of the possibility for a transfer. Of course this is best done in advance.

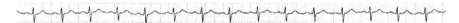

8 The Case of Truth: A Conference on Defensive Medicine

Physician's Perspective

I was going to a continuous medical education conference. All physicians are required to have continuous medical education, but the definition of what is education has been broadening. I will speak more about this in the chapter entitled *The Medical Industry and Medicalization*. Here I will give one specific example. This was a full day conference required by the malpractice insurance carrier. How can malpractice insurance impose an educational requirement? By providing a discount of thousands of dollars for those who will attend. The cost of a medical malpractice insurance for a family physician practicing obstetrics in my part of the country is $37,000 per year! The conference had a politically correct name of improving quality of patient care. The goal of the conference in fact was to reduce costs associated with medical malpractice lawsuits. Quality of care is not always related to the amount of money that can be lost as a result of lawsuits. While I dreaded going to this conference, I found the information interesting.

Societal Perspective

Some lectures were presented by lawyers. The lawyers spoke to us about the importance of documentation. They told us that when it comes to a lawsuit, the truth is irretrievable and unimportant. Only facts that are available at the time of the investigation are important. The job of the lawyer on each side is to convince the jury of his version of the truth. Documentation, or to be more precise, defensive documentation, is what is important. Hence the doctors and nurses spend a third to more than a half of their time maintaining medical records. What was originally done for the purpose of communication about the patient's condition is now done also for protection against lawsuits and for the justification of insurance billing.

Physicians who are employed by the malpractice insurance company also lectured and educated us. We were told that most awards after a successful lawsuit in obstetrics are given for *delay to C-section*. The strategy then was to increase the rate of C-sections, thus removing the possibility of a delay. The nationwide appeal to reduce the C-section rate is a sham. To reassure us, we were shown data that after 32 weeks the newborn's survival does not change much (normal gestation is 40 weeks). They tried to convince us that there is no need to try to wait till term, instead, C-section should be performed at the first sign of trouble. This was hard for me to believe, so I went up to the speaker at the end of the lecture to ask him how reliable this data was. He reassured me that it was totally reliable, that the only difficulties with the more premature newborns were difficulties feeding and maintaining body temperature, but survival was unchanged. No information was given on the longer term consequences. The point was that, at the first sign of trouble after 32 weeks gestation, one is justified in performing a C-section. To reduce losses, we are supposed to reduce the threshold for C-sections. That was the bottom line.

A year later I received an invitation to a follow up risk management lecture. This time the incentive was not large and the institution for which I work did not oblige me to go to this Continuing Medical Education (CME) event, see Figs. 7-2 and 7-3. Such 'educational' activities are not sporadic; they are systematic and well organized. Such 'educational' methods are designed to maintain a defensive state of mind in a physician thus protecting the insurance company.

Other specialists shared other tricks of dealing with the litigious system. We were presented with the idea of using a system design similar to one used in the *aviation industry*. Aviation has a system of redundant checks where a possibility for a mistake is eliminated in most cases. There is always a second pilot present, for example, to monitor the first. The airplane is also monitored from the ground. The pilot cannot make a deviation from the course because his autonomy is very limited. Hospitals throughout the US are now implementing similar principles into medicine. The future will show whether this system works. The result of this model is a more uniform approach with less likelihood of deviating from the course. While in some cases this will surely prevent errors, it also makes medicine more mechanical. I mean mechanical in a sense that actions take place automatically as if done by a machine. My feeling is that this movement was initiated by the hospitals throughout the country as a means of protecting themselves from lawsuits, but as usually, under a politically correct name of *risk management and quality improvement*. Physicians lose some degree of autonomy as do patients. We hope that in the majority of cases it will be for their own good, but we don't know if that will be so.

Medicine seems to be more complex than piloting an airplane, needing more flexibility and the ability to change the course according to individual needs. The course of medical policy is determined by the authorities who create guidelines. These authorities, as we all, are prone to making a mistake. Though such mistakes may be less frequent, they are likely to produce more far reaching consequences than a mistake by a single doctor. They can also be influenced by the industry which has the power of indirect bribing (as will be illustrated in the chapter entitled *Medical Industry and Medicalization*), and skewing study results to their advantage.

Here is what happens in practice at the hospital (it has already begun). When a patient, say with an exacerbation of heart failure, enters the hospital, there are pre-printed forms indicating what should be ordered. If a physician does not follow the form he has to explain why. The explanation better be good in case he ends up in court. The pre-printed forms are but the first level of this defense. Later along the pathway, the nurses are being trained to question physicians when a certain pre-determined pathway is not followed. While there is a pretense of developing teamwork skills, the nurses are specifically trained to be the monitors and recorders (often in the form of incident reports) of doctor's decisions and unfavorable outcomes. This has created more doctor-nurse tensions. Further, the hospital trains the nurses in so called high risk areas (such as obstetrics) to remind physicians of the need for a consultation with a specialist when there are troubles. Nurses are obliged to make reports of all that is unusual or not going well. Why this is done will soon become more apparent. The third line of protection is formed by the various "quality control" committees that collect data on the physicians to identify the "high risk" physicians. High risk in this case means the risk of a lawsuit that will cost the hospital a lot of money. With the help of the documentation, the hospital then can get rid of such a liability. There are numerous consequences of this system to the health care providers and to the patients. It increases conflicts between doctors and nurses. The nurses are forced to be part of the enforcement system which generally they don't like being.

Patient/Family Perspective

The doctors and the patients lose autonomy. In a large hospital, any deviation from the standard protocols will be met with significant resistance. For instance, if a mother would wish that her newborn child would not get the antibacterial ointment into its eyes and an injection of Vitamin

K, she can no longer refuse. The automatic pilot of the system will have taken over, freedom of choice is lost.

Physician's Perspective

Below is an example of an order form for congestive heart failure exacerbation (Fig. 7-1) that's used in one hospital. It is generally helpful because many aspects of care have been thought through and mentioned here, so they won't be accidentally overlooked. Here you may also notice a subtle enforcement tool. Under medications, if a doctor did not check the first two medications he then has to explain himself in the "If not, why?" section. In this particular instance, one should not have much trouble explaining. This form, however, illustrates a trend, that if continued too far will take more and more autonomy from both doctors and patients. In the hospital where I work, there are more than ten such forms available and new forms are being developed. They cover less acute and non-pathological conditions such as neonatal jaundice (usually a normal slight yellowing of the skin of the newborn baby in the first week of life) and childbirth.

When a certain condition (such as neonatal jaundice) is encountered, the patient falls into the hospital protocol for repeated blood level measurements and treatments based on those levels. All this is automatic. While it is said that a doctor can always override the protocol, very few doctors are willing to expose themselves to such risks, and few will actually give it a thought after getting used to it. Hospital practice of medicine is becoming more mechanical (as is outpatient practice) so that a patient who enters the system and the doctor practicing in it are passive implementers of the guidelines.

Fig. 7-1: Pre-printed physician's orders for Congestive Heart Failure

PLEASE WRITE FIRMLY USING BLACK BALL POINT PEN

■ UNLESS THIS BOX IS CHECKED, A FORMULARY EQUIVALENT MEDICATION MAY BE SUBSTITUTED BY PHARMACY

ALL LISTED ORDERS ARE IN EFFECT UNLESS CROSSED OUT. EXCEPTIONS: ORDERS PRECEDED BY A BOX (☐)
REQUIRES A (√) TO INITIATE. ORDERS WITH BLANKS INDICATE ADDITIONAL INFORMATION IS NEEDED.

PATIENT NAME		AGE	SEX	PHYSICIAN	ADMITTING DIAGNOSIS
DATE	TIME		ALLERGIES/INTOLERANCES		

ADMIT STATUS:　☐ INPATIENT　　☐ OUTPATIENT　　☐ OBSERVATION

1. Admit to:　☐ Progressive Care Unit　☐ Medical Floor　☐ ICU
2. Baseline heart failure stage (see reverse):_____
3. Weigh patient on admission and then each and every day. Record in kg.
4. Strict I&O q shift
5. Diet:　☐ Reg　☐ NAS　☐ 2 gm Na　☐ Low Fat/Low Cholesterol　☐ ADA _____ Cal.
   　　　☐ Full liquid　☐ Clear Liquid　☐ NPO　☐ Other_____
6. ☐ Fluid restriction 1 1.5 2 liters/day (circle choice)
7. ☐ Insert Foley
8. Code Status:　☐ Full Code　　☐ No Code　　☐ Limited Code _____　☐ Not established
9. Labs on admission (unless performed in ED):　☐ CBC　☐ CMP　☐ TSH　☐ CKMB　☐ Troponin　☐ BNP
   　　　　　　　　　　　　　　　　　☐ Digoxin level　☐ Mg　☐ Other:_____
10. Labs in AM following admission:　☐ CBC　☐ BMP　☐ CKMB Q 6 hrs.　☐ Troponin　Other:_____
11. ECG on admission and PRN chest pain.　QAM x _____ days
12. CXR on admission:　☐ PA/Lat　☐ Portable upright (if not done in the ED)
13. Respiratory therapy:　☐ Oximetry　☐ Oxygen @ _____ L/min. per NC to maintain SaO2 . 90%
   　　　　　　　　　　　☐ Nebulizer per protocol or:_____
14. Smoking cessation counseling (ACC Class I Indicator* if patient has smoked within the last 12 months)
   　☐ Nicotine replacement per Pharmacy protocol
15. Vital signs: ☐ Routine Other:_____
16. Notify UM Nurse to ensure that patient's ejection fraction is recorded in chart (ACC Class I Indicator*)
17. If previous ejection fraction cannot be obtained by the physician or the resource nurse within 24 hours, obtain
   echocardiogram (ACC Class I Indicator*)
18. IV diuretics on admission_____　IV:_____ mg　Q_____ hr after ED dosing.
   　　　　　　　　　　(Drug Name)　　　(Dose)
   ☐ If urine output less than 250cc within 2 hours, give double the dose IV to maximum of_____ mg.
19. Sliding scale potassium:　☐ Oral (PTCA) scale　☐ IV (CV) scale
20. MEDICATIONS (see reverse side for medications information)
   ☐ ACE or ARB:_____ If not, why? _____ (ACC Class I Indicator*)
   ☐ Beta Blocker:_____ If not, why? _____ (ACC Class I Indicator*)
   ☐ Spironolactone_____　☐ ASA: 80 mg QD
   ☐ Digoxin_____　☐ Acetaminophen: 650 mg Q 4-6 hours PRN mild pain
   ☐ LES PRN
21. Activity: ☐ As tolerated　☐ Bedrest　☐ BSC　☐ Chair　☐ Ambulate x_____ /day
22. Referrals:　☐ Social Services　☐ Nutrition Services　☐ Outpatient follow-up - SHIP/SHAPES

* American College of Cardiology Class I Indicator: Conditions for which there is evidence and/or general agreement that a given
procedure or treatment is useful and effective.

PATIENT LABEL

409890 (5/03)

X _____
(VALID ONLY WHEN SIGNED BY PHYSICIAN)

REGIONAL HEALTH SERVICES

HEART FAILURE ORDERS

Fig. 7-2: Invitation to a CME Program

Insurance Company

2965 Ryan Drive S.E. • Salem, Oregon 97301-8074 • (503) 371-8228 • toll-free 1-800-243-3503
P.O. Box 13400 • Salem, Oregon 97309-1400 • FAX (503) 371-0087 • www.npmic.com

V O U C H E R → VALUE OF $50

Exclusively for Policyholders of Northwest Physicians Mutual Insurance Company

This non-transferable voucher is for:
Reznik, Oleg

NPM Policy #:
6201.014

This voucher is valid towards attendance at the following program:

Practicing Medicine in a Changing Environment:
Addressing Patient Safety, Medical Malpractice and Risk Management
Friday, December 10, 2004
Multnomah Athletic Club, Portland, Oregon

If you plan to attend, you may use this $50 voucher to reduce your registration fee from $195 to $145. Attach this voucher to your completed registration form (located in the enclosed brochure) along with payment and mail to: TFME, One SW Columbia St., Suite 860, Portland, OR 97258. DO NOT SEND TO NPM.

✂ ═══

October 13, 2004

℃ß

Dear Policyholder:

You're invited to attend the 16th Annual Regional Symposium presented by The Foundation for Medical Excellence (TFME) in cooperation with Northwest Physicians Mutual (NPM). We have enclosed the brochure about this program for your consideration.

Your attendance will qualify for NPM Loss Prevention Workshop (LPW) premium discount. TFME also designates this educational activity for a maximum of 6 Category 1 credits towards the AMA Physician's Recognition Award. The Oregon State Bar has approved this course for 6.25 hours general CLE credits.

Questions regarding your LPW status? ☎ Amy Bielenberg at NPM (800-243-3503).
Questions regarding the program? ☎ TFME, Portland, OR (503-636-2234).

One needs to know that the incentive here is not a mere $50.00 but the fact that this course is accepted as a continuous medical education which is required of all physicians annually in order to maintain their board certification.

Fig. 7-3: Invitation to a CME Program.

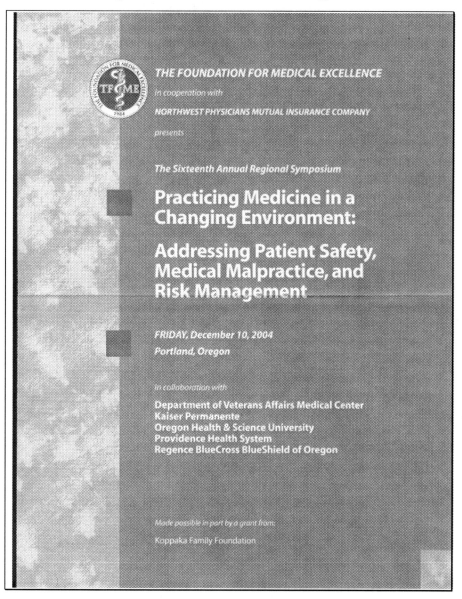

Risk management, of course, is a politically correct name for *how to avoid a lawsuit*. Patient safety as well as the idea that the foundation proposing it is truly for medical excellence is a sham, only safety from a lawsuit is considered. As I mentioned earlier at the initial conference we were encourage to increase the rate of C-sections so that the delay to C-section as a major source of money loss would be eliminated.

In the outpatient sphere, this automatization is driven primarily, and possibly inadvertently by the medical industry, which enforces its will by influencing medical guidelines, medical education, and indirectly medical malpractice law.

A story from my last year of residency can illustrate this point. As I mentioned, my residency program was at a university hospital. That usually means that a more academic/scientific approach to teaching is emphasized. Nevertheless, about half of the speakers who lectured the residents were "sponsored" by the pharmaceutical companies. This was a lecture presented to us by a big expert on cholesterol, someone who published articles on the topic in the major journals. A lecture hall was full with residents and faculty. He taught us about the new stricter guidelines for treating high cholesterol. He was "sponsored" by a pharmaceutical company that made one of the new, expensive and powerful combination drugs for lowering cholesterol. This was the second change of guidelines during my training that called for treatment with medications for still lower levels of cholesterol. The speaker was explaining to us how important it was to be aggressive with treatment, that we would be saving people from heart attacks and strokes. I was in for a surprise when I asked him whether there were data on total mortality (data that showed that people who took that medication ended up living longer, not just had fewer heart attacks). Admittedly, this type of data are hard to come by. It was not his answer that surprised me but the manner in which he responded. He became visibly angry and raised his voice. He said that this kind of data is difficult to obtain (not a surprise) but that if he were an expert witness on a plaintiff's side after a plaintiff had a heart attack and I (and he pointed his finger at me from the podium) did not treat this plaintiff according to these guidelines, he would "tear me up to shreds." Following was a moment of silence, and I could sense fear spread throughout the big lecture hall. He then went on to complete his lecture and showed the slides provided to him by the pharmaceutical company.

Now I'll go over this case, showing how each of the three whips of the medical industry (the guidelines, the education, and the law) are played out. We will go over the **guidelines** in greater detail in the chapter entitled *Medical Industry and Medicalization.* For now, I would like to say only that the majority of clinical trials are industry sponsored. There are multiple ways of manipulating the results of the studies by altering study design, statistical analysis, and reporting of results. This is the way the guidelines are manipulated. What confirms my suspicion is that the guidelines of other western countries are less strict for blood pressure, cholesterol, and blood sugar than those of the US.

The example above clearly shows the influence on the medical malpractice law. The big shot doctor was threatening to "tear me up to shreds" if I did not comply. Naturally, a doctor cannot tell his patient—you should take this medication because I am afraid of being torn up to shreds in court. Instead, a doctor feels forced to resort to other techniques of persuasion. He'll often resort to subtle threats. When he does not succeed, he deems patient non-compliant.

Patient/Family Perspective

Overall I would recommend to the patient never to react to fear. If a doctor makes you feel afraid, recognize it as a signal not to follow his advice, and smile.

Physician's Perspective

With respect to **medical education,** I would like to clarify what it means for a doctor to be sponsored by a pharmaceutical company. It means that the pharmaceutical company will pay the speaker $400-1500 for a lecture, depending on the number of people expected to attend, prestige of the institution where the lecture will be given, and prestige of the lecturer. The company then makes an agreement with the speaker that he'll use at least a certain number of slides in his presentation that are provided by the pharmaceutical company, and/or emphasize a drug made by the sponsors. Naturally, this is designed to promote the latest and most expensive product (older products run out of patent and are no longer big money makers). As we all know, pharmaceuticals also have an extensive direct-to-consumer advertising campaign in the media. There is also advertising suggesting that we are always on the brink of discovering a new and life-saving treatment for any number of illnesses, hence trying to obtain the newest product becomes very important to the consumer (the patients) since this may be the cure and the end of suffering as implied but not overtly stated in the advertising. This theme plays on the emotions of patients who are suffering of a serious illness and who believe that the medical system will relieve them of this suffering.

In a residency program, faculty members are not supposed to solicit residents to pharmaceutical-sponsored dinners given by them. This would mean that they were using their position for making additional money by promoting a pharmaceutical product. Dinners are another way physicians are educated by the pharmaceuticals. Your meal at a nice restaurant is paid for by the pharmaceutical company, and a company sponsored lecturer teaches you. Fig. 7- 5 on the following pages illustrates one of the many invitations to such dinners that I and every physician receives in mail. The money offered by the pharmaceuticals becomes a temptation. Few will pass up making an easy additional $1000 per month. I encountered one faculty member during my residency, who found his way of profiting from the pharmaceutical companies. His wife was not a faculty member, but she was a specialist (hence an expert in certain aspects of medicine). She became the speaker at the pharmaceutical dinners and he solicited residents to attend it. No one was technically breaking the rules, but he and his wife made the money. I show this example to illustrate again the influence of money, and the "creativity" that it can inspire in people. The lecture would have a politically correct name such as Advances in Management of Disease "X", but emphasis would be placed on one or two recently produced drugs. The result of this for the patient is promulgation of treatments that are unnecessary, expensive, and sometimes harmful.

Fig. 7-4: A letter from a drug representative, addressed to me.

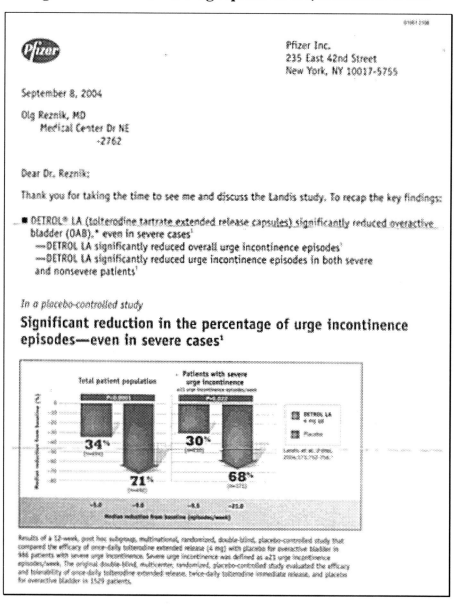

I did not ask for this information and I did not take the time to discuss the so-called 'Landis study', as the letter is stating. The drug representative did stop by to drop off some medication samples in the organization that employs me. It is another trick to keep the name of the product in the physician's mind.

Fig. 7-5: An "expert" lecture sponsored by a pharmaceutical company.

Customizing Care
FOR THE Menopausal Woman

Donna   , MD

Professor of OB/GYN at the University of Southern California

Estrogen Therapy

J. James Restaurant
325 High St. SE
Pringle Park Plaza
Salem, OR 97301
503-362-0888

Wednesday September 22, 2004

Reception at 6:30 PM

Dinner at 7:00 PM

Please RSVP by Monday, September 20, leaving Name and

Phone Number with Michele Feeley @ 503-551-3982 or Dave

Homma @ 503-620-8048

This program is sponsored by Wyeth Pharmaceuticals. The purpose of this program is to
educate health care professionals about issues related to menopause and Wyeth products.
It is inappropriate to invite or pay for spouses or guests to attend Wyeth-sponsored
Visiting Speaker's Bureau (VSB) events.

 Wyeth

© 2004, Wyeth Pharmaceuticals Inc., Philadelphia PA 19101 February 2004   107734-03

One of many invitations every physician receives in the mail.

Fig. 7-6: A lecture by another expert sponsored by the company that manufactures product.

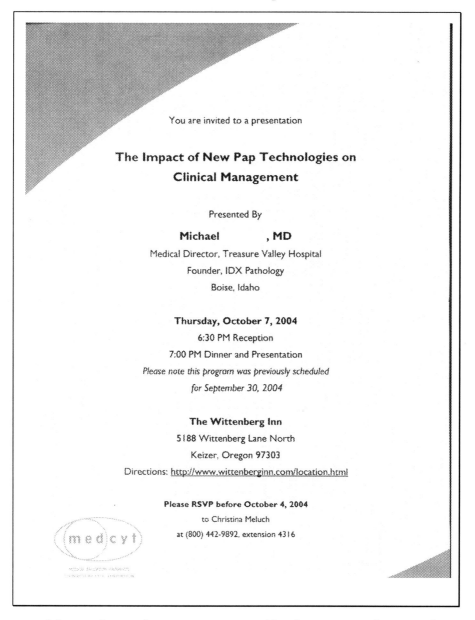

You are invited to a presentation

The Impact of New Pap Technologies on Clinical Management

Presented By

Michael   , MD

Medical Director, Treasure Valley Hospital

Founder, IDX Pathology

Boise, Idaho

Thursday, October 7, 2004

6:30 PM Reception

7:00 PM Dinner and Presentation

Please note this program was previously scheduled

for September 30, 2004

The Wittenberg Inn

5188 Wittenberg Lane North

Keizer, Oregon 97303

Directions: http://www.wittenberginn.com/location.html

Please RSVP before October 4, 2004

to Christina Meluch

at (800) 442-9892, extension 4316

med)cyt

A lecture by another expert sponsored by the company that manufactures product (the new Pap smear technology) that is being promoted.

Fig. 7-7: An invitation for a CME dinner

You are cordially invited to attend
an interactive presentation on

Getting it Right the First Time: Early and Effective Treatment of Major Depressive Disorder

Presented by

Charles   , MD

Associate Clinical Professor of Psychiatry
Tulane University School of Medicine
Louisiana State University School of Medicine

J. James Restaurant
325 High Street SE, Salem, OR 97302
Call 1-503-362-0888 for Directions

Thursday, October 21st
6:30 PM

Please **RSVP** to Dave Homa
(503)-475-2017

Wyeth®

The purpose of this program is to provide health care professionals with information about Wyeth products and the disease states treated by these products. Therefore, it is against Wyeth policy to invite or pay for spouses or guests to attend Wyeth-sponsored Visiting Speaker Bureau (VSB) events.

© 2004, Wyeth Pharmaceuticals, Inc., Philadelphia, PA 19101. 169889-02 October 2004

Of particular interest in this invitation is the fact that the physician offering the lecture is a faculty member at a medical school, hence involved in training of medical students and residents. As one can see, he is also sponsored by one of the big pharmaceutical companies and, without a doubt, the talk will try to encourage prescribing of the drugs produced by this company.

Physician's Perspective

It is hard for a physician to overcome this biasing of medical information. Under the pressure of time, the physician will prescribe the first medication that comes to his mind, when treating any given medical problem. I know this from personal experience. The drug representatives' job is to keep the names of the drugs they sell in the physicians' minds.

Patient/Family Perspective

It is even harder to overcome this biasing for the patient. Most patients, as do most physicians, do not verify the information they receive from the pharmaceuticals. The patients receive their information through the bias of the direct-to-consumer advertising on TV and other media.

How can the patient tackle the issue of bias and automatization in medical care? Regarding a hospital setting, it is best, of course, to avoid getting hospitalized altogether. If one has to enter the hospital system, smaller hospitals may be more accommodating but may not have all the specialists and procedures available at large hospitals. In a large hospital, one needs to be actively involved in medical decisions and have the courage to refuse tests and treatments that are offered, when they do not seem justified. A physician will feel much more comfortable if he can write down that a patient refuses a certain treatment. Performing tests or treatments on a patient who does not wish to have them is assault and battery.

In an outpatient setting, one must be wary when feeling pressured by the doctor to take a certain medication or undergo a certain procedure. This pressure does not mean that the doctor is evil. He may simply not have enough time to provide the education, or may be fearful of legal repercussions from not following guidelines. Nevertheless, since the possibility of harm exists with almost any medical treatment, I believe a physician never has the right to pressure a patient. The physician's job is to present options, make recommendations and answer questions.

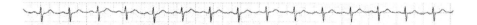

9 The Case of a Quiet Rebel

Patient/Family Perspective

This was a fifty-six year old man with an advanced lung cancer that was discovered recently, and congestive heart failure that he had been known to have for a few years prior to his hospitalization. He was admitted to the hospital because of pneumonia. He was also anemic and his kidneys had begun to fail. I was at the end of my internship, working under the supervision of a senior resident and an attending physician. When I made my morning rounds, the patient was quiet and calm. He did not appear depressed and answered a few routine questions I asked him. An intern almost never has the time to have a meaningful conversation with a patient. In addition to pneumonia (an infiltrate that was seen on chest CT), he also had some fluid next to his lung (pleural effusion).

We started him on the stronger antibiotics, some intravenous fluid, oxygen, nebulized breathing treatments. So far he accepted everything without objections after asking us few questions about our findings. Our attending physician, seeing that patient's condition was complex, asked us to obtain a cardiology, pulmonology, and nephrology consults (There is no shortage of consultants at a university hospital).

Physician's Perspective

My senior and I happened to be of a similar mind set. By philosophy we were both non-interventionists (doctors who prefer to do nothing when the benefit of an intervention is not clear). We were both aware of the limitations of a medical system in this case. A person with the type of lung cancer this patient had could not be helped very much. The available data showed that with chemotherapy, his life would be prolonged by an average of seventy-eight days (two to three months) and that, if he were treated with chemotherapy, he would likely experience some toxic effects. This is hardly a bargain. Nevertheless, seventy eight days is considered to be a statistically significant difference (Agra et al., 2003). Hence, the pulmonologist was very surprised when the patient stated that he preferred not to treat his cancer with chemotherapy. Outside the patient's room, I cautiously inquired about the reasons for treatment and expressed my impression that life was not prolonged by much. The pulmonologist responded that while that was true, to him it seemed that the people who were treated appeared healthier until they died and those not treated faded away gradually. That did not make much sense to me since chemotherapy has side-effects that can make one quite sick.

Patient/Family Perspective

The patient then proceeded to refuse a chest tube placement recommended by a pulmonologist to remove the fluid around the lung, and blood transfusions mentioned by the kidney doctor.

Physician's Perspective

When the team (our attending physician, senior resident, and an intern—myself) went into the room, we were supposed to say what the specialists recommended. We could not say what our opinion was unless the patient asked, and even then I am not sure whether we would have had the courage to recommend against the specialist's opinion in front of our attending physician. The patient did not ask for our opinion. He simply said that he didn't want to have those treatments and procedures. Our attending physician then added a few things to try to convince the patient to accept the procedures. He seemed to believe that the patient should have everything that the specialists recommended.

I felt that the patient's decisions were appropriate and was reassured when my senior resident told me that that he was thrilled that the patient was refusing everything. We quietly shared this satisfaction until the patient's pneumonia improved and he went home with a home hospice program. The patient never found out that two doctors in the room always agreed with his decisions. I will try to explain why we (my senior resident and I) were happy about patient's decisions and why we did not speak up.

Patient/Family Perspective

It is far more common to see the opposite: the patient who eagerly and desperately grabs onto every straw thrown by the doctors. A patient may undergo futile tests and treatments, suffering more from that than he would have, by refusing. When appropriate, refusal of treatment helps to preserve one's dignity and prevents one from turning into a test object. The pulmonologist who offered chemotherapy was not an evil person. He was following his guidelines. Maybe he had even looked at a study, and a study says that the difference between treatment and no treatment is statistically significant, hence it makes a difference even though the difference is very small.

The pulmonologist is actually used to patients who want everything done even if there is a minutest chance of improvement, used to patients who believe that medicine has all the answers. So the pulmonologist offers what he can, which in this case is not much at all. The patient then has to decide for himself since it is his life on the line. The patient needs to ask questions that would help him decide. The doctor then has to answer honestly, if he knows the answer, or admit ignorance if he doesn't know.

Physician's Perspective

We were happy about the patient's refusal of treatment because we didn't have to participate in something that caused unjustified suffering. It seemed unjustified to us, but it may not always seem unjustified to the patient. Since it is the patient's life on the line we try not to make decisions for him. Because he did not ask for our opinion, quite appropriately we did not offer it. If he had asked, we would have had to gather enough courage to give an opinion that was different from that of our attending physician.

Patient/Family Perspective

This patient was not passive, he did accept a short treatment for pneumonia, but did not want to accept anything more drastic. I think he had asked his questions before and was set on what he wanted before he entered the hospital. Sometimes new and surprising findings in the hospital prompt one to reconsider his prior decisions. If your mind is set, don't doubt yourself and don't ask for opinions that you don't need. If you are in the process of decision making and need information, don't be afraid to ask whether what you want to do is reasonable. From the answers, you'll usually know what to do. If the reasons given by the doctor don't seem important to you, if you sense that the doctor is pressuring you or appealing to fear, the answer is usually to do the opposite of the recommendation. Be your own authority, or you become someone else's agenda.

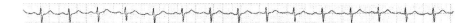

10 The Cases of a Compliant and Not So Compliant Surrender

Patient/Family Perspective

This was a sixty year old woman who one day decided to see a doctor because of feeling tired and noticing a big lump on her breast. Her physician realized after examining her that this was likely to be cancer. She lived in a rural area, so her doctor sent her to see a specialist in a town about one hour away. After some investigative studies, a diagnosis of a metastatic breast cancer was made. This woman was a relative of my wife. She was surprised by the diagnosis since no one else in her family had any kind of cancer. She was advised to have surgery, chemotherapy, and radiation. She did not question any of the proposed therapies, completely trusting that the doctors would know best what to do. After a mastectomy with lymph node resection, her arm became swollen. Her life had changed drastically as she now had to go to a nearby town for regular treatments of chemotherapy and radiation. She was experiencing side-effects of treatments. This went on for two years.

One day, she woke up extremely short of breath. She was taken to the hospital where it was found that she had a pulmonary embolism. It is a known and very dangerous condition that can be caused, among many other things, by cancer. She was receiving blood transfusions because chemotherapy made her very anemic. Fluid was now accumulating in her lungs and she needed procedures to remove that fluid. After the pulmonary embolism, she was told that she could go to a subacute facility, where treatments would continue, or she could now give up therapy. She felt that at this point giving up would mean that all those two years of suffering and therapy were for nothing. This was the first time she was given a real choice, and she chose to continue treatment. She was weak, short of breath, and in pain due to a combination of factors, both illness-related, and treatment-related. When she passed away, one of the doctors told the family that the treatment had probably been futile. They were disturbed to find that out. They did not sue. I was not involved directly or indirectly in her care. I also found it disturbing that a doctor who administered the treatments found them futile but never told that to the patient. The patient trusted that the doctor would do what was best for her.

In my second year of residency, I saw a patient whose response to the news of cancer was not typical. An elderly couple came to see me because the man was coughing and feeling progressively worsening shortness of breath. As I spoke to them more, I found out that he used to be a smoker of many years and quit smoking when his elder son died of lung cancer at age forty-five, five years earlier. The man was now seventy-five years old. He was calm and quiet and his wife tended to give a lot more details in response to my questions. She was visibly anxious about her husband's condition. She reported that his appetite has worsened and that he was starting to lose weight. His physical exam was unremarkable. I sent him for an X-ray and pulmonary function tests. X-ray came back suggestive of a mass the size of a plum. CT scan confirmed that he had now several adjacent masses in his left lung and one in the right. I described the findings to them.

Physician's Perspective

It was my first time to give someone news of advanced cancer. I looked up the statistics, but did not speak about survival until they asked me. His wife was calmer than on the first visit. It seemed that she knew. The patient was as calm as at his initial visit. They then asked me about "his chances". I told him that this varies depending on the stage and the type of cancer, and that it was impossible to predict for each particular individual, but that if he wanted I could give him the "averages". He did want to hear it, and I read off to him, from a page I'd printed out earlier, the percentages of five year survival for several different stages of several different types of lung cancer. I gave them the page to look over and keep. They listened with mild interest, and did not react as if I was telling something too important. Then I automatically proceeded to do what I was trained to do—tell that they needed a referral to pulmonologist who would be the appropriate specialist to manage the problem. In retrospect, I recognized that this was a mistake, and I was glad that they did not follow my initial suggestion. Instead of providing information and finding out about their preferences, I initially proceeded along the mechanical, pre-determined, non-individualized algorhithm.

Patient/Family Perspective

Their roles seemed to change. The wife who spoke a lot during the first visit was now quiet. The husband said, "Well, we'll take your referral paper and think about it." I was taken by surprise and, to be sure that they understood the urgency of the situation, told them that this process may progress rapidly. The wife then told me a story of their elder son who lived close to them and whose struggle and death they'd witnessed. It seemed their son's cancer was diagnosed at a similar stage. He then went through surgery and six months of chemotherapy with radiation. He was sick from the treatments. His life revolved around his therapy. He was always coming or going to some treatment and had less time than before to spend with his own family. Then he died.

The husband (the patient) now said that he did not want to go through the same. We left it at that, and I didn't hear from them until his wife came accompanying one of their grandchildren whom I was to see for a school physical. She told me that her husband died at home about three months before. She said he was in peace.

Physician's Perspective

Some time after, when I was in my third year of residency, I encountered another patient for whom our team uncovered the diagnosis of cancer. This was a forty-eight year old man who came to ER because of swelling and pain in his leg that had been worsening over the previous several weeks.

We thought that this was a blood clot (deep venous thrombosis—DVT). He did not have signs of infection, but his leg felt strange, not like the usual DVT, but wood-like. Repeated studies showed that there was no clot but the condition was not improving. Finally a biopsy showed a rare form of cancer. It was a metastasis, but with all the investigations we never found the source, which is not uncommon. By this time a number of consultants were involved.

Patient/Family Perspective

The patient was a married man who in the past overcame an addiction, worked, and loved fishing. He would tell me about his fishing experiences, as I was an appreciative listener and used to fish a lot while I was growing up. We both truly enjoyed his stories.

The time came for him to be discharged. He was set up for radiation and chemotherapy treatments. Specialists also recommended discharging him with a medication that prevents blood clots, but can cause bleeding as a side-effect. I continued visiting him even when it was another doctor's turn to do hospital work. As I said goodbye on the day of his discharge, he asked me what I thought of him going fishing. He was concerned because our attending physician advised him not to fish because of the risk of bleeding. I told him that there was that risk, but that I did not think that would stop me if I was in his situation. He smiled.

A month later, a medical student who was also involved in this patient's care and stayed in touch with the patient and his family told me that he had passed away, but he did go fishing.

I present these stories not to discourage people from seeking medical treatments but to have a more realistic outlook. On a daily basis we are bombarded by suggestions from the media that imply medical omnipotence. I will address this in more detail in the chapter entitled *Illusions of Medical Omnipotence*. For now, I would like to show that passivity on the side of the patient is not likely to be helpful for that patient. In fact there is even some scientific data suggesting that people with an *active coping style,* those who are actively involved in making medical decisions about their care, do better when it comes to deadly disease (Faller et al, 2002).

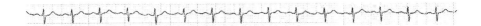

11 Ulysses Syndrome and the Case of the Endless Search for Reassurance

Societal Perspective

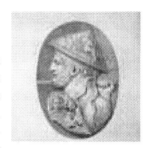

Ulysses (in Latin), also known as Odysseus (in Greek), is the main hero of Homer's *Odyssey*. He was one of the Greek kings who fought in the Trojan War against the Trojans. It took him twenty years to return home, and his travels described in the Odyssey were beset by many hardships.

If you look up the definition of Ulysses Syndrome in a medical dictionary, you will find: The ill effects of extensive diagnostic investigations conducted because of a false-positive result in the course of routine laboratory screening; or: ill effects from follow-up diagnostic tests following a false-positive screening test. The term was first coined by the Canadian physician Dr. Mercer Rang. Just like Ulysses, today's patient is in danger of embarking on a journey that brings more suffering than he had to begin with and from which it may take him a long time to return. A cascade of unnecessary tests and procedures can be set off by a false positive test.

This syndrome is now on the rise as we do more and more screening tests. The usual screening tests such as screening mammography, prostate cancer screening, colorectal cancer screening and some of the prenatal screening tests can lead to it. Ulysses syndrome can also occur after almost any test you get unless you are prepared to accept some risk and to stop the endless search for personal reassurance from your doctor.

Patient/Family Perspective

I could cite many examples, as this is a frequently recurring theme. A patient came to me for sinusitis, and as this was her initial visit, I inquired about other health problems. This was a fifty-eight year old woman without any significant past medical history. She was a librarian, a mother of two healthy children who were now grown. She lived with her husband and still worked full time. After hearing a radio commercial, she was persuaded to go to one of those CT scans that were supposed to identify coronary disease. She was worried about her heart because of occasional unexplained chest pains. She was not satisfied when her prior physician told her that her chest pains were not from her heart after she had a negative stress test. A chest X-ray was normal. A trial of a medication for heartburn did not help. The self-paid CT scan showed no significant heart disease, but incidentally discovered a nodule in her lung.

She had never smoked and had no family history of cancer; nevertheless she could not ignore this. She went to see a pulmonologist and was now in the *pulmonary nodule clinic*. This clinic was specially designed for patients with incidentally discovered nodules in the lungs. And there were many. Doctors in than clinic collected all prior CT scans of each patient, and reviewed them to check for enlargement every six months. Every six months, she had a repeat CT scan of the affected region to verify whether or not the nodule was growing. She said she was supposed to do that for two years or else get it resected which would be difficult and posed more risks. By the time I met her she had only one more CT scan to go, but she shared how unsettling it felt to just let this nodule sit there, knowing that this "could be a potential time-bomb."

Physician's Perspective

Several things that I chose not to share with her ran through my mind. One was the risk of cancer related to repeat exposure to radiation from CT scans. Not many people are aware that a CT scan (of the chest) exposes one to at least one hundred times the radiation of a chest X-ray (Reuter et al., 2002). Another was how her wish to get reassurance by obtaining a study that she hoped would give her a solid diagnosis, something one can hung one's hat on, resulted in a much less reassuring situation. She said she continued to experience occasional chest pains but they were no longer the focus of her attention. Her physical examination confirmed her sinusitis, and we said goodbye after I gave her prescription for the antibiotic she desired.

A similar situation occurred just a week before I started writing this chapter. On one of the usual days at the office I saw one of our medical assistants silently crying in the corner. I inquired gently. She replied she had a head CT scan and it came back abnormal. It turned out she saw one of my partners for her migraines. A well meaning doctor ordered a head CT, which showed an abnormality at the base of the skull versus an artifact. Artifact is an abnormal finding due to the limitations or malfunctions of the testing equipment, not a true abnormality. CT scans are known to create those at the base of the skull, because the bones in that region are particularly dense. With mental agony she waited for a week to get an MRI (a more accurate study in this case) which came back normal.

I see at least one patient per week with a similar dilemma. They have a symptom that has not been explained by tests, and their response is a wish to do more tests. The certainty of discovering a deadly illness is preferred to the uncertainty of not knowing what the symptom may mean. Patients told me many times that they would have preferred to know what they had no matter how dangerous it may be rather then accept uncertainty.

Societal Perspective

This theme ties into the belief in medical omnipotence and will be discussed more in the chapter dedicated to that topic. I cannot blame a patient for such beliefs. The media is constantly suggesting that we are progressing and overcoming great illnesses. If you pay attention to this advertising, you will notice that almost always it is tied up to someone making a profit. It may be an appeal to contribute money for research, or a suggestion that we should go and be screened for a certain illness. Often innocent and famous people get caught up in this and will be endorsing it on TV. Such were the campaigns of truly well meaning and altruistic women to popularize and to teach other women breast self exam in order to discover early breast cancer and prevent its progression. It was not too long ago. It is an intervention that is no longer routinely recommended. Two large well conducted studies showed that breast self exam leads to unnecessary breast biopsies, but does not result in saving lives. As a result of these findings, even a conservative agency, such as United States Preventive Services Task Force, now states: "The USPSTF concludes that the evidence is insufficient to recommend for or against teaching or per-forming routine breast self-examination" (USPSTF, February 2002). This happened in 2002, after many years of teaching and performing it. Promotions for breast self exam were based on ideas, as opposed to empirical evidence, and turned out to be harmful to women but helpful to those who reaped financial benefits of the additional unnecessary biopsies and follow up visits.

Partly because of our innate discomfort with uncertainty and to a large degree because of the suggestions we receive from the media and the medical system, we tend to have an unreasonable expectation about the capabilities of medicine. We expect that a test result will bring certainty by establishing a definitive diagnosis. We believe that if it is negative we are secure about not getting an illness in the foreseeable future. We believe that if we follow the guidelines offered by the medical system we are safe. And, we believe that treatments offered by today's medicine usually provide permanent solutions. All these are false beliefs.

Patient/Family Perspective

I advise my loved ones to know when to stop and not be caught up in the *Ulysses Syndrome* type of journey. We don't need a journey accompanied by more suffering than we originally tried to avoid, nor do we need unnecessary tests, procedures, and side-effects. Some time ago, my mother asked me to give her advice on what to do about her slightly abnormal mammogram. With the information that I knew about her, I advised her never to go back to repeat it. There was some risk, but I thought it was justified. My mother chose to follow my advice and did not go back. So far, six and a half years later, she is well. A question may come up, will you still think your advice was good if she develops breast cancer? The answer is yes. The test is not very good, and its usefulness in low risk people is questionable (as will be discussed in the chapter entitled *It is OK to Hurt Many a Little in Order to Prevent One From Getting Hurt a Lot*). It is a mistake to think that by getting a test you are guaranteed not to get an illness, as it is naïve to believe that omitting a test causes one to get sick. In addition, the hope that if the cancer is discovered earlier the woman will live significantly longer, has not been substantiated by evidence (as will be discussed in the chapter entitled *Illusions of Medical Omnipotence*).

Physician's Perspective

A very illustrative case is a description of one doctor's own saga, which he published in a professional newsletter (Kopes-Kerr, 2004). After an episode of rectal bleeding in 1988, he went for a colonoscopy. During this procedure, after cleansing the colon with purgative medications, a flexible scope is advanced through the anus about six feet, until the entire colon is visualized. After a day of "miserable preparation protocol, and losing another day to the procedure" he learned that for technical reasons colonoscopy could not be performed all the way. The scope which normally is advanced to the full length of the colon could not be passed beyond the initial one third. This is an important point to be aware of. Any procedure can unexpectedly run into some technical difficulty. The specialist told this patient that there were no abnormalities in the part that he was able to look at.

In 2002, this patient/doctor had another episode of rectal bleeding. He went to a different gastroenterologist who also performed a colonoscopy. Again this man went through a day of preparation and lost another day to the procedure. Again the specialist was not able to go beyond the same point about a third of the way up. This time, however, in the part that he saw, he discovered and removed a polyp that turned out to be pre-cancerous. The specialist did not recommend trying another colonoscopy because of the limitation of the procedure. Because of the particular anatomy of the patient, another attempt would only expose the patient to additional risk of perforating his colon. Instead the specialist recommended "virtual colonoscopy" (computed tomographic colonography). After preparation, the colon is pumped up with air, then a CT scan is performed.

Insurance did not cover this expensive and still experimental procedure. It was not available at the hospital where the patient worked. During a delay created by the circumstances, some major scientific data came out questioning the usefulness of virtual colonoscopy. It misses a lot of lesions, and for those that are not missed, it does not tell what they are. Dr. Kopes-Kerr writes: "What would I do if they saw a small "something"? We are talking about a laparotomy (open surgical procedure to explore the colon directly) with possible partial colectomy (removal of part of the colon). All this for what may be nothing? And if this year's test is negative, they'll want to do one next year. And so on. Forever. I don't think so."

The story demonstrates another very important point—"Ask what will be next; what will we do with the results." It is a mistake for a patient to assume that their doctor will have thought it through. Dr. Kopes-Kerr realized virtual colonoscopy was unreliable. It is a poor test that is likely to generate some abnormal result. The next step then would have been surgery, a major surgery with general anesthesia that may result in removing a part of his intestine. Since virtual colonoscopy cannot distinguish between benign and malignant polyps, an unjustified surgery could have been done. Benign polyps need not be removed, they are harmless.

Patient/Family Perspective

The most important point here in my opinion was his ability to stop. He says, "Now I have to live with the thought that maybe I do have more proximal polyps (polyps in the area that was not seen during colonoscopy), and maybe they too have high grade dysplasia (pre-cancerous). This would imply a fairly significant risk of colon cancer. What do I do? My answer is to let fate play its hand. I am not interested in a major abdominal procedure "just in case". I am going to die of something, maybe sooner than later, and it is likely to be either heart disease or cancer. So why not colon cancer?"

Of course this is an academic physician, who is a residency program director and a publisher of a brilliant professional literature review. He is also a courageous human being whom I witnessed apply his courage in his care of patients as in this case he is applying it to himself. But you can not expect this from your usual doctor. If they told you that it's not worth it for you to have a certain test, they would be exposing themselves to risk. They are aware that there is always some chance that you'll have a certain illness or maybe even die. They fear that you (the patient) or your family will sue them, if later you develop an illness that at least in theory could have been detected by that test, and at least in theory, prevented from progressing. Unfortunately, neither detection nor prevention are guaranteed by tests. The risk of a lawsuit seems too great to the vast majority of doctors. Lots of tests of this kind are performed every day, costing a lot of money and sometimes resulting in harm to the patient. For those reasons, I believe that in our health care system the patient has to take the initiative about a decision to stop. It is all right not to have a certain test to begin with or to stop having more and more tests to reassure oneself or the physician that the possibly abnormal result is not really abnormal. No amount of testing can prevent you from getting sick; no amount of testing can prevent you from dying. You, the patient, need to take the active role, decide when to test and when to stop testing.

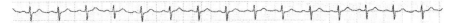

12 The Case of Insurance Casualty and a Sense of Entitlement

Patient/Family Perspective

While in the previous chapter I tried to address the issue of stopping additional unnecessary testing, here I will talk about the issue of starting tests for the wrong reasons to begin with. A fifty-seven year old woman came to me with her husband to establish care. They had recently moved from another state. She'd never worked; they had several grown children. She told me that she has a good insurance and she wanted "everything done." She literally wanted to do as many tests and consultations as possible, believing that this would bring her good health. She did have high blood pressure and was taking a medication for it. I am always wary with a patient like this and from the beginning try to establish how much I'll have to give into her demands without causing her much harm or driving her away. We started with the usual. I went over her need for a screening mammography and colorectal cancer screening, Pap smear, and went on to a flu vaccine and blood tests. She did not have chest pains, reportedly her cholesterol was normal, she had never smoked, and she had no significant family history. She apparently read a lot on the internet, and told me that she wanted to be tested for diabetes and thyroid dysfunction. I did not object, reserving my protests for what I sensed was coming later. She wanted an ECG but did not mention a stress test, and I had a silent sigh of relief. The sticking point turned out to be the timing of a Pap smear.

Physician's Perspective

This woman has had annual Pap smears since she was twenty one. She told me that she'd never had an abnormal Pap smear, or a sexually transmitted disease. She'd been married for thirty three years. Her last Pap smear was one year ago and she wanted to set one up right away. I then told her that the recommendations on the frequency of Pap smears have changed. For women who never had an abnormal Pap smear and had at least three pap smears, annual testing is not necessary. Testing once in three years is sufficient. She appeared troubled, and I went on to say that, as an example, for women older then sixty five without past abnormalities, there is no evidence to support screening at all, because of the increased risks of false-positive results and invasive procedures (USPSTF, February 6, 2003). More frequent screening in her case would increase her risk for having a false positive result without providing any additional benefit.

The patient now started to look at me with some suspicion. I think she felt that I was trying to cheat her out of some of her insurance benefits. She then told me that she had fibroids (benign tumors of the uterus) and wished to go to a GYN specialist to discuss the issue of Pap smear with him and also to discuss surgery for her fibroids. The patient said these fibroids were incidentally discovered on the ultrasound that she'd had a few years prior for an episode of vaginal bleeding. At that time she also had a biopsy of the inside of her uterus and everything was normal. I told her that the fibroids were not dangerous and, when they are not too bothersome, the surgery is not necessary. She only continued to look at me with suspicion and repeated her request for a GYN consultation. By that time I had already gone way beyond the time allotted for the visit, and agreed to do everything as she requested without further discussion.

Patient/Family Perspective

Soon after, I received a consultation note from the gynecologist. She (the gynecologist) advised the patient not to have a surgery for fibroids, but did perform a Pap smear. I could not blame her, since the patient who is insistent about getting a test or a procedure that is covered by the insurance will almost always get it. The Pap smear came up slightly abnormal. The patient was given a short course of local hormonal treatment, and a Pap smear was repeated in a few months. It came back slightly abnormal again "atypical squamous cells of unknown significance" (ASCUS) and the patient was set up to have a colposcopy with biopsy. Colposcopy is a procedure in which a doctor looks at the cervix (the opening of the uterus) with an instrument that illuminates and magnifies. Certain chemicals are applied, making abnormal tissues more visible and, when necessary, biopsy is performed. Biopsy turned out to be normal but as a "precaution" she was told to return for repeat pap smears every six months for the next two years. She continued to see me for the management of her high blood pressure. We did not discuss the progress of her gynecological treatments, but she seemed to trust me more as the time went on. I was glad she didn't end up losing her uterus unnecessarily. As for her endless Pap smears, I knew they were not likely to amount to anything except an additional thing to worry about for the next two years.

I was hoping she would initiate the conversation and ask for my opinion on the need to continue these procedures, but she never did.

The situation described here can occur with any patient, but it reaches its maximal harm in those with good health insurance. I have seen patients who have had multiple procedures and surgery as a result of their request to be tested for everything. Passing up on a test sometimes seems to the patient like being cheated out of something they are entitled to, something that is paid for by the insurance. This is not surprising to me. One of the reasons is that while the need for Pap smears is widely advertised, the link with the sexually transmitted nature of the disease we are trying to screen for is not well publicized. Most women who come to me for colposcopy after being referred for abnormal Pap smear are surprised to learn that the cervical cancer that we screen for is caused almost exclusively by a sexually transmitted virus (human papilloma virus—HPV). In fact, I recently performed a Pap smear on a seventy five year old woman who has not been sexually active for more than a decade, simply because I could not talk her out of it. She insisted that she wouldn't have peace of mind without it. I was greatly relieved that it came back completely normal.

Health insurance can be a double-edged sword, damaging those who do not realize that tests are not harmless. When my loved ones ask, I give advice determined by their baseline risk. In medicine this is called a 'pre-test probability' and means, to put it simply, how likely are you to have a disease that you are trying to test for. There are very few tests for very few specific problems that give 100% correct answer 100% of the time. None of the screening tests can do that, and even the invasive diagnostic tests are not 100% accurate. The less likely you are to have the disease you are testing for, the more likely you are to get a false positive result and be caught by the *Ulysses Syndrome*.

There is a time to ask an important question. After your doctor does his interview and physical examination, you may be asked to undergo some initial tests. When the results come back, he may want more tests. At that stage, ask, "How likely am I to have whatever it is we are testing for." If the answer is not very likely but we'd rather be "safe than sorry", it is very rarely a good idea to proceed with testing. Just stopping and accepting some uncertainty and some possibility of disease and death will almost always save one from additional unnecessary suffering. I would caution against the so called routine tests. If you are feeling well and living a healthy lifestyle, the need for any routine test is questionable. If you are inactive, obese, addicted to cigarettes, drugs, or alcohol, emotionally distraught, or unable to manage your animal drives, then there are things to do, and you know what to do for most of those things without the help of a doctor. The most effective preventive care is one done by the patient himself by altering these simple lifestyle choices. A routine visit to a doctor can perhaps increase awareness about one's unhealthy choices. Few or no tests are necessary for that.

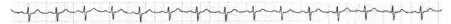

13 The Medical Model

Societal Perspective

Much of the material in this chapter comes from an article "The End of the Disease Era" recently published in *The American Journal of Medicine* (Tinetti, 2004), and some discussion will go beyond the scope of the article. The article talks essentially about the inadequacy of the current medical model in addressing health problems of today's patient. It also explores some alternatives. Awareness of this can help the patient understand why their doctors press them to take a large number of medications for the rest of their lives. This article also describes how the current model leads to undertreatment, overtreatment, and mistreatment of patients.

The current medical model, as it is taught in medical schools and practiced, is based on treatment of acute diseases. It is disease-oriented. "When disease became the focus of Western medicine in the 19th and early 20th century, the average life-expectancy was 47 years and most clinical encounters were for acute illness. Today, the average life-expectancy in developed countries is seventy four years and increasing, and most clinical encounters are for chronic illness or nondisease-specific complaints."

Hippocrates said "Tell me not what disease the patient has, but what patient has a disease."

Physician's Perspective

The current medical model has departed far from this view of health and illness. Today, physicians are taught for the most part that it doesn't matter who the patient is (what kind of human being they are, what is important to them), instead the focus is on understanding the disease—a set of findings that fits a certain label. Once this label is placed, we treat the label by following predetermined algorithms with minimal inter-individual variations. Physicians are trained and encouraged to treat the disease, not the person, nor the symptom.

Patient/Family Perspective

This, however, is not always helpful for the patient. For example, the patient who comes to seek help for dizziness undergoes a number of tests to figure out what disease is causing it. If the disease (anemia, low blood pressure, inflammation of the inner ear, insufficiency of certain blood vessels in the brain, certain type of a migraine, a metabolic problem, a drug, etc.) is not found, more often then not the patient will be told that nothing is wrong. Sometimes the implication is that the patient is crazy, and no treatment maybe offered. The authors of the article mention some of the problems that this approach engenders. "Chronic dizziness (and many other symptoms that cannot be assigned to a specific disease label) remains unrelieved; psychological contributors to cardiovascular disease are ignored; 75-year old patients consume an average of 15 medication doses each day; patients leave the hospital with their pneumonia cured but their cognitive and physical function irreversibly impaired."

Societal Perspective

Healthy people are also subject to multiple recommendations. "Decision making for relatively healthy adults is governed at present by a litany of recommended behaviors (e.g. smoking cessation, safe sex, increased physical activity, and decreased alcohol intake); preventive services (e.g. mammography, colonoscopy, regular dental care, bone mineral density measurement, immunization); and, depending on age, sex, genetic predisposition, and screening results, daily use of medications such as aspirin, statins (cholesterol lowering drugs), calcium, vitamin D, and bisphosphonates (osteoporosis drugs) which are all predicated on preventing specific diseases."

Spiritual/Philosophical Perspective

The disease-oriented model results in inappropriate treatment because it follows predetermined protocols centered on treatment of a specific disease, and ignores the patient's nature. The following paragraph represents my own views, though I believe the authors of the article would agree.

The disease model is based on the belief in randomness. It stems from the idea that life was created by an accident or a succession of random events that brought a new level of organization. As an extension of this human beings are seen as mechanical organisms subjugated to the laws of randomness, cause and effect, and entropy. Disease is believed to result from the effect of randomness on the "nature and nurture" complex. For example, one can be born with genes that predispose one to high blood pressure, this is nature. One then is immersed into the environment that makes his blood pressure more likely to rise (poor diet, stress)—this is nurture. Genetic predisposition becomes manifest as a disease when the environment pushes one over a certain threshold, the threshold that is varied and ruled by chance. The randomness is essential here and is more easily seen in the studies done on identical twins. Such twins have identical sets of genes and very similar environments, yet one will get a disease and another won't. This difference is believed to be due to chance. More broadly, when one smoker will get lung cancer and another won't, the afflicted person is essentially told that it's his bad luck. You will often experience this when you ask your doctor about the reason you have a certain illness. The usual answer is—no one knows (with an implication that it happened by chance). In the model based on randomness, consciousness is seen as a mere extension of the highly organized matter—the brain. This is one of the main reasons that the contribution of mind to health and illness is ignored or minimized. The idea that emotional, mental, moral, and spiritual aspects of a human being may be fundamental in developing and maintaining health is difficult to even consider for one whose thinking is rooted in randomness and meaninglessness of existence.

Patient/Family Perspective

In the above mentioned article the authors give several examples of *undertreatment* due to being confined to this model. Treatment for depressive symptoms may be withheld when a patient does not meet all the criteria of the Diagnostic Statistical Manual (DSM-IV)—the diagnostic bible of psychiatry. Chronic dizziness and chronic non-cancer pain that result from the interplay of treatable physical and psychological factors will often be left unalleviated when the diagnostic workup does not reveal a "causative" disease. "Undertreatment also occurs in 'traditional' disease categories such as coronary artery disease. A wealth of data links cardiovascular outcomes to socioeconomic, psychological, and environmental factors, as well as to biological determinants. Despite compelling evidence of the effectiveness of interventions such as antidepressants and counseling, clinical attention remains primarily targeted on the use of beta-blockers, lipid-lowering drugs, and other such treatments. Treating only the biological mechanisms—an offshoot of the focus on disease—rather than addressing all contributing factors results in lost opportunities to maximize health outcomes."

Overtreatment is seen in aggressively treating the very elderly and demented patients to the point of having them experience the side-effects of treatments or in heroic attempts to keep alive multiply-handicapped very premature babies, brain damaged accident survivors, and terminal cancer sufferers. Overtreatment is routinely seen in nursing homes. The authors also give an example of a "70 year old patient who suffers from an average of four chronic diseases in addition to nondisease-specific health conditions such as pain, impaired mobility, and disordered sleep. The emphasis on diagnosing and treating individual diseases has led to a plethora of disease management guidelines. For example, for a patient with the not uncommon combination of diabetes, heart failure, myocardial infarction, hypertension and osteoporosis to comply with existing guidelines, a physician must prescribe up to 15 medications." Taking such a large number of medications increases the risks of adverse effects and drug interactions resulting in more adverse effects. For instance, a recent study found that patients taking the antibiotic erythromycin had twofold increase in the risk of sudden cardiac death because it interacts with many other medications (Ray et al., 2004).

I would also add that there are no studies on the particular combinations of diseases. They don't exist simply because it would be too hard to find enough patients with the exact same set of diseases and study them. So, while the benefits of these drugs were proven for some of the individual conditions, it is much less clear whether treating someone with all the drugs recommended for each individual disease at the same time is of benefit. I would not be too surprised, if it turned out to be harmful after you reach a certain number of medications, simply because of the higher chance of adverse effects. The long term use of these medications worsens the problem. One of my patients comes to mind because she happens to have a very similar set of conditions as described above. She is a sixty two year old woman with diabetes, hypertension, myocardial infarction and heart failure, plus she is mildly mentally retarded. She comes to see me accompanied by her guardian. After I'd put her on most but not all medications required by the guidelines, she told me that "It's too many pills and I won't take any more than what I'm taking." Her guardian was somewhat embarrassed by what seemed like irresponsible or unintelligent behavior. For legal reasons, in my chart note, I described this and labeled her with poor adherence. Later I wondered, however, whether her mental retardation allowed her to make a smarter choice in the long run than one made by most physicians and patients.

In the article, the authors describe *mistreatment* as an unintentional result of ignoring patient preferences and making clinical decisions solely on disease-specific outcomes. "Patients vary in the importance they place on survival, comfort, and functioning, and in the choices they make when faced with difficult tradeoffs. Hospitals are filled with patients whose infection or organ failure "responded" to up-to-date technology but whose physical, cognitive, and psychological functioning deteriorated." I couldn't agree more.

I remember attending a patient with advanced lung cancer that metastasized to the brain. At that time, I was a registered nurse working at the hospital part time while attending pre-med at New York University. From the orthopedic floor where I usually worked, I was floated to oncology to substitute for another nurse. The patient was a man in his early fifties. He could no longer respond when spoken to because of the brain involvement. Nevertheless, he would open his eyes, and no one knew whether he was still aware of what was going on. I knew, however, that he was aware of pain. His cancer treatment caused elevated blood sugars. My job as a nurse was among other things to check his blood sugars every two hours and administer insulin, if required. I remember clearly the sound of suffering that came out of him every time I punctured the skin on his finger with a lancet in order to obtain a drop of blood. His whole body shook as if in a small convulsion. Neither his family nor his doctors were there to witness this, over and over again. From this and other experiences as a nurse I learned to pay attention to nurses' reports and opinions. What I had to do did not make sense to me but I continued to carry out duties that were imposed on me. Several weeks later I learned of that patient's death in the hospital. When his mind gave out and he was no longer able to make decisions about his own care, the family designated all of the decision-making to the doctor. Most likely the doctor mechanically did what he was trained and asked to do—everything. So everything was done to this patient before he died. As it turned out in this case, doing everything was not in his best interest. Doing everything increased his suffering but did not increase either length or quality of his life. One could say that this patient was unintentionally but severely mistreated.

Physician's Perspective

Doctors given inordinate responsibility are usually unable to exercise it to the patient's best interest. Previous chapters have covered some of the reasons: fear of a lawsuit, guidelines and treatment algorithms asking for certain treatments and monitoring tests for a generic patient with a certain condition, training that does not emphasize that patient preferences are valuable, lack of time to see and reflect on what the patient is going through.

Societal Perspective

In the article, the authors' proposed solution is to create an individualized approach. With that approach, treatment would be guided by the "patient's articulation of preferred trade-offs between long-term outcomes such as survival and functioning and short term acceptance of testing burden, lifestyle changes, and the inconvenience, costs, and side-effects of daily medications." The authors proposed that the concept of the individual disease be integrated into individually tailored care.

It seems like a very sound recommendation to me. It is time-consuming to try to find out what is important for the patient. Perhaps more time and money would become available if we didn't automatically try to do everything for everybody. Among many barriers to the individually tailored care is the fact that "the transition... will require a major reorganization of health care from education through delivery system." As it appears to me, the *individually tailored care model* proposed by the authors would be a great deal more flexible and would accommodate health views held by a variety of patients. It would, for example, allow for non-chance based models of health to be integrated into health care. Mind, meaning and spirituality could be added to body in an integral way, and used as guiding principles when treating a patient who finds addressing these aspects valuable. Patients would be treated with more dignity and would have a chance of becoming their own authorities and taking responsibility for their health which in itself is a step toward health that they are usually denied at present.

Finally, this approach would save a great deal of money that's now being spent on forcing multiple lifetime medications on most patients, then monitoring and treating side-effects. This money would probably be better spent on the social programs that increase the quality of life of the poorest in this country, which in return would further reduce health care costs in addition to providing much needed help. While sophisticated devices such as a mechanical heart pump (left ventricular assist device (LVAD), and new pills get the most attention in the media, it is not what truly saves lives. Instead, it is very simple measures such as improving living conditions, hygiene, and education that prevent most health problems.

Patient/Family Perspective

For a patient navigating through the health care system now, I would recommend again not to give up authority to the doctor. In cases where you feel undertreated, or blown off as not having a problem, or implied that you are crazy, try the following. Say that you understand that a specific disease causing your symptom was not found. Nevertheless, since you experience the symptom, you'd like to have some sort of treatment to try to make it better. If there are no conventional treatments, inquire about alternative ones. Hopefully, that'll get you the help you need. Nowadays, there are various forms of alternative treatments that are holistic and not necessarily 'unsicentific'. Changing a doctor may be necessary sometimes, but don't get into an endless cycle of doctor shopping. Usually, non-confrontational inquiry in the manner I presented will help the doctor to shift his or her thinking from trying to treat the disease to treating a symptom that troubles you.

In the case of overtreatment, and this is the case when doctor tries to impose a treatment that seems excessive to you based on your personal preferences, say to the doctor that you understand that the guidelines for treating your disease require more or higher doses of the medication, but your personal preference is not to take it. Tell the doctor (after finding out) that you understand the risks involved and are willing to accept them. Do not be afraid of being judged as irresponsible or unintelligent. Do not be afraid to state that the inconvenience of taking more pills, or of having to get regular blood tests, or of the possibility of side effects and interactions etc. are not worth it for you. Start getting used to the idea that your personal preferences are important. Do not take the pill to please your doctor or lie about having taken it. Most doctors will be OK treating a patient "suboptimally" if the patient understands and accepts the risks involved with this "suboptimal" treatment.

The cases of mistreatment often happen when patients are either not able to make decisions as in dementia or advanced disease, or give carte blanche to the doctor to make all decisions for them. Because of the conflicts of interest that I described above, not many doctors are actually able to act in patient's best interest. It is a challenge to the best of physicians. I believe that the patient or family must accept and exercise the responsibility of decision-making. They must not be shy about expressing their preferences, about asking questions, and must not be too concerned about what someone else will think, but rather articulate their preferences openly and clearly.

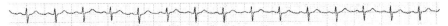

14 The Medical Industry and Medicalization

Societal Perspective

The medical industry is one of the most powerful industries worldwide and exerts an enormous influence on the way medicine is practiced as well as the direction of future developments. On the one hand it has provided us with medications, devices and treatments that are lifesaving. On the other hand, it is responsible, to a large degree, for rising healthcare costs and mistreatment of patients by influencing the dynamic of several processes guiding medical care in the US. The medical industry influences medical education through pharmaceutically sponsored lecturing. It influences practice guidelines through manipulation of scientific research, which for the most part is pharmaceutically sponsored. It drives the process of 'medicalization'—a process whereby the threshold for what is considered abnormal is continuously lowered creating more and more customers for lifetime medical treatments. The term medicalization first appeared in *Medical Nemesis* by Ivan Illich. It is achieved by directing research to show that people with lower levels of certain markers such as for example blood pressure, cholesterol, blood sugar, live longer. Research is directed through sponsorship—a pharmaceutical offering money to study a specific topic. A leap of faith then is usually made to say that if we lower these markers in any person, that person will live longer. In some cases this may be true. The company then will make a drug that lowers these markers; the guiding agencies are prompted by the research to alter guidelines. Most patients and some doctors are unaware of this dynamic. The patients are surprised to find out from their doctor that they are "supposed" to take more and more medications for the rest of their lives.

An example of this kind of occurrence can be traced by looking at a recent story with hormone replacement therapy (HRT) for post-menopausal women. For many women, menopause brings the discomfort of hot flashes, increased risk of osteoporosis, and more heart disease. The industry realized that it can make a product—a hormone replacement pill. There was an idea that since women start having more heart attacks after entering a menopause, perhaps hormones are protective against heart disease, in addition to helping with osteoporosis and hot flashes. Then *observational* studies were done which showed that hormones indeed seemed protective against heart disease. The guidelines were immediately created to say that postmenopausal women should take HRT, and millions of women throughout the world were encouraged to do so from the time of the menopause and for the rest of their lives. One needs to ask oneself, what is an observational study and what can it tell us. It cannot tell cause and effect but tells only of a correlation. I can observe that the sun rises soon after I put on my slippers in the morning. This however does not mean that my act of putting on of slippers causes sunrise. It turned out that the conclusions of the observational study were wrong because the women that were looked at were overall healthier and more health-conscious then the women they were compared with. When a randomized clinical trial compared similar women, those who got HRT had more problems (more heart attacks and slightly more breast cancer). Findings of these studies brought the current downfall of HRT.

There is now a new HRT—low-dose estrogen patch for osteoporosis. The drug seems to increase bone density but it's not known yet whether it will prevent fractures. To know that takes time. It also takes time to know whether it's safer than the original HRT. The idea of this patch may sound nice until you find out that a woman with a uterus (who hasn't had a hysterectomy) should undergo an endometrial biopsy at least once a year while on this drug, to monitor for development of a precancerous condition (The Medical Letter, 2004). Endometrial biopsy is not a pleasant procedure and is not without side-effects.

Industry also distorts the data by using a variety of means. Statistical manipulation of data, publication bias, emphasizing relative but not absolute risks are but a few examples. A well known example of a publication bias was discovered in 2001 with a study on Celebrex (Silverstein et al, 2000). The pharmaceutical company obtained results that showed less gastrointestinal side-effects (when compared with a much cheaper ibuprofen) at six months but no difference at twelve months. They chose to publish (in the Journal of American Medical Association—JAMA) the six months result but withheld the twelve months result, thus creating an illusion of a far superior drug. "JAMA's editor, Catherine D. DeAngelis, said the journal's editors were not informed about the missing data. "I am disheartened to hear that they had those data at the time that they submitted [the manuscript] to us," she said. "We are functioning on a level of trust that was, perhaps, broken." (Okie, 2001). This was one example that probably is a tiniest tip of a huge iceberg.

The experts in the guiding agencies are not always free of bias. For the specialists, stricter guidelines usually mean more referrals and more business as the primary care physicians are bound to be quickly overwhelmed by the rising numbers of the customers—patients needing treatments. In fact, specialty groups often create research to suggest that screening for more diseases is necessary. If the idea is accepted, the primary care physician is then given the role of a case finder—someone who finds cases and refers them to the specialist. This process is not inherently evil, but only becomes so when financial interests outweigh the altruistic ones. In a recent article, a group of vascular surgeons were urging primary care physicians to increase awareness of peripheral arterial disease, and to initiate screening protocols for patients at higher risk for this condition (Belch, 2003). Peripheral artery disease is a narrowing of the arteries supplying legs that is similar to narrowing of the arteries of the heart that leads to heart attacks. It causes pain in calves while walking. The recommendation is in the face of the fact that there are no data to support such a screening program, meaning that there is nothing to suggest that discovering peripheral arterial disease in patients who have no symptoms is going to help these patients. Once the condition is discovered by a screening test, further testing would have to be done and this further testing is invasive and can cause harm. The patients would then be labeled with having a disease, implying the need for treatment, which in this case is of no benefit for the patient. Such a screening program on the other hand would send a lot of business into the hands of the vascular surgeons.

Another example is given by another recent study that tries to encourage more investigation to find ovarian cancer (Goff et al., 2004). It offers a questionnaire type of scoring system for assessing symptoms and recommends to do further diagnostic investigation to those who screen positive. They admit that 8% of women presenting to primary care clinic will screen positive. So, if one was to follow their recommendation, he'd have to investigate 8% of women, even though the incidence of ovarian cancer in the US is 16 per 100,000. This means that for every one woman with ovarian cancer, more than four hundred women without cancer would have to undergo an investigation for suspected ovarian cancer, the cancer that even when found, is not very treatable. As I keep mentioning, testing in itself is almost never benign because it can lead to unnecessary procedures, complications, and mental anguish from being labeled with a disease. Imagine those more than four hundred women who would spend weeks and maybe months thinking that they may have cancer, and undergoing investigative procedures and surgery to find out in the end that all this was unnecessary.

Medicalization is a trend of lowering the threshold for what is considered medically abnormal and hence constitutes a disease and requires treatment. It is seen particularly clearly when one looks at the trends in guidelines with respect to blood pressure, blood sugar and cholesterol. The new guidelines for hypertension, for example, came up with a new category that is called pre-hypertension (JNC-VII, 2003) (systolic blood pressure 120-140, and diastolic 80-90). These numbers were considered normal in the previous guidelines. According to the new guidelines, one needs to make lifestyle changes when in that range and start taking pills when above it, without exceptions. This puts a lot of people on pills. In contrast, the British, who have access to the same data, continue reasserting that for low risk people medication does not need to be prescribed until blood pressure is above 160 systolic and 100 diastolic (Williams et al., 2004).

Similarly, the guidelines for blood sugar have changed. In 2002, the guideline producers—HHS and ADA—released a statement warning Americans of the risks of "pre-diabetes"(Prescriber's Letter 2002). This was probably done with the good intention of prompting people to take preventive steps. What followed was a slew of studies showing how taking some drugs preventively will protect you from developing diabetes as effectively as lifestyle changes. There are now at least two drugs that are regularly prescribed for pre-diabetics (Chiasson et al., 2002; Diabetes Prevention Program Research Group, 2002). Patients are given a suggestion that the pill is a way of escaping the need to change. One needs not change one's lifestyle, all one needs to do is take another pill for life.

Moving on to cholesterol, in this area the guidelines seem to change every year and now there is no longer a threshold below which you are OK. The guidelines now say that if you are at high risk for heart disease, the lower your cholesterol, the better. In the new guidelines for people with heart disease, one must start taking a drug for cholesterol if LDL is higher than 100 (the old threshold was 130), while the goal for the "very high risk" patients has dropped to less than 70 (Grundy et al., 2004). When reading these guidelines, one may begin to equate heart disease with cholesterol. In reality, cholesterol is one of the numerous components that influence heart health, many of the others are still unknown. An example of this lack of scientific understanding of heart disease comes from the issue of hormone replacement therapy again. Women who took hormones had better cholesterol. This was thought to be one of the reasons that hormones would protect the heart. As we had seen that didn't happen. In the new guidelines for the use of Hormone Replacement Therapy, an expert says: "…medical experts may have overestimated the effect of cholesterol in heart health, and been unaware of other factors in heart disease that we still don't understand" (ACOG News release Sept. 30, 2004).

Why were the prior cholesterol guidelines made more stringent? The panel of experts responds, "Updating of the Adult Treatment Panel III (ATP III) guidelines (which were the prior guidelines) was initiated because recent clinical trials had provided evidence regarding several significant issues pertaining to the benefits of cholesterol lowering." You may find reading the financial disclosure of this panel interesting:

ATP III Update 2004: Financial Disclosure.

Dr. Grundy has received honoraria from Merck, Pfizer, Sankyo, Bayer, Merck/Schering-Plough, Kos, Abbott, Bristol-Myers Squibb, and AstraZeneca; he has received research grants from Merck, Abbott, and Glaxo Smith Kline.

Dr. Cleeman has no financial relationships to disclose.

Dr. Bairey Merz has received lecture honoraria from Pfizer, Merck, and Kos; she has served as a consultant for Pfizer, Bayer, and EHC (Merck); she has received unrestricted institutional grants for Continuing Medical Education from Pfizer, Procter & Gamble, Novartis, Wyeth, AstraZeneca, and Bristol-Myers Squibb Medical Imaging; she has received a research grant from Merck; she has stock in Boston Scientific, IVAX, Eli Lilly, Medtronic, Johnson & Johnson, SCIPIE Insurance, ATS Medical, and Biosite.

Dr. Brewer has received honoraria from AstraZeneca, Pfizer, Lipid Sciences, Merck, Merck/Schering-Plough, Fournier, Tularik, Esperion, and Novartis; he has served as a consultant for AstraZeneca, Pfizer, Lipid Sciences, Merck, Merck/Schering-Plough, Fournier, Tularik, Sankyo, and Novartis.

Dr. Clark has received honoraria for educational presentations from Abbott, AstraZeneca, Bristol-Myers Squibb, Merck, and Pfizer; he has received grant/research support from Abbott, AstraZeneca, Bristol-Myers Squibb, Merck, and Pfizer.

Dr. Hunninghake has received honoraria for consulting and speakers bureau from AstraZeneca, Merck, Merck/Schering-Plough, and Pfizer, and for consulting from Kos; he has received research grants from AstraZeneca, Bristol-Myers Squibb, Kos, Merck, Merck/Schering-Plough, Novartis, and Pfizer.

Dr. Pasternak has served as a speaker for Pfizer, Merck, Merck/Schering-Plough, Takeda, Kos, BMS-Sanofi, and Novartis; he has served as a consultant for Merck, Merck/Schering-Plough, Sanofi, Pfizer Health Solutions, Johnson & Johnson-Merck, and AstraZeneca.

Dr. Smith has received institutional research support from Merck; he has stock in Medtronic and Johnson & Johnson.

Dr. Stone has received honoraria for educational lectures from Abbott, AstraZeneca, Bristol-Myers Squibb, Kos, Merck, Merck/Schering-Plough, Novartis, Pfizer, Reliant, and Sankyo; he has served as a consultant for Abbott, Merck, Merck/Schering-Plough, Pfizer, and Reliant.

All of this can be found on the National Institute of Health website[1].

The new guidelines guarantee that more people will be placed on cholesterol lowering medications, that the dosages of the medications will be higher, and that people will be on the medications longer. The validity of the need for this change is debated by many individuals and organizations, including Center for Science in the Public Interest. While cholesterol lowering drugs have their place in medicine, extremes are likely to be harmful.

Patient/Family Perspective

How do we deal with all this? First, I would recommend some healthy skepticism. The idea that medical care will make you immortal is false. "The exciting new drug" has almost always turned out not to be so exciting, given time. There is a side-effect to almost every drug or treatment. When a doctor is proposing you to take more medications, ask some questions that would help you determine whether this is something for you. If you are OK with the risk of the side effects and inconveniences involved and find that the benefit is worthwhile, then by all means take the drug. Be aware, though, that what is believed to be good today may be found harmful tomorrow even if the greatest of authorities are endorsing

---

[1] See http://www.nhlbi.nih.gov/guidelines/cholesterol/atp3upd04_disclose.htm

it now; remember that one hundred years ago almost none of the drugs we use today existed. Someone may be tempted to say that we live a lot longer now because of the modern medicine, but this is only partially true. Improvements in sanitary conditions are responsible for most of the longevity increase; people living to be one hundred years old and more is not a phenomenon unique to this century. After reading a draft of this chapter, Dr. Bob Rich, a psychologist, writer, and friend added, "…length of life is only one consideration. Living life popping pills and worrying about every little twinge is a lot inferior to robust activity that ignores discomfort. Life is about meaning, not illusory safety."

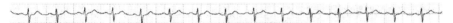

15

It is OK to Hurt Many a Little in Order to Prevent One From Getting Hurt a Lot

Societal Perspective

At first, this seems reasonable to a health professional. We are trained about the importance of screening and immunization and how they work. When we speak of populations, all seems well, but when it comes to the individual, no one wants to be the one to get hurt unnecessarily. The definition of what is unnecessary varies from one person to another. While immunization, at least in theory, has the potential of helping the many, the story with widespread screening is not as straightforward. My reason for bringing up this issue is to tackle the idea that the authorities know better. This idea is a remnant of the older paternalistic system that belongs in the past. The authorities do not always know best.

Recently, a flu vaccine manufacturer had to suspend production and distribution of the vaccine because it was contaminated (AAFP This Week, 10/5/04). Can someone guarantee that none of the vaccines distributed before were contaminated? The answer is no. In addition, a vaccine has side-effects. If you've heard people say that they got a flu from the vaccine, they are not far from the truth. In medical language it is called an oculo-respiratory syndrome. Though not as severe as a flu, it is like catching a cold and you can get it from the flu vaccine (Skowronski et al., 2003).

Physician's Perspective

Immunization and screening tests are often insisted upon by doctors in order to comply with the guidelines and to pass the audit of the insurance companies. I say 'insisted' because the doctor is placed into a position of having a vested interest in patients undergoing all the recommended screening procedures. When in this position, often without realizing it, he will try to persuade the patient by fear tactics. A doctor is in a position of a great influence, which makes it a very privileged position. The doctor is in a position to threaten the patient with death by mentioning the possible deadly outcomes of not screening. Because of the bias, the doctor is also less likely to talk about the downsides of screening such as two in a thousand risk of colon perforation with colonoscopy, the 18% chance of getting an unnecessary biopsy with ten years of mammography screening, and the lack of proven benefit from prostate cancer screening at all (USPSTF 2002). To clarify this, a screening test is a test done on a patient who feels fine and who has no symptoms (otherwise it would be called a 'diagnostic' test not screening test). It is done with the hope of discovering a disease before it produces symptoms. The thinking is that at an early stage the disease is more treatable or more likely to be cured.

Societal Perspective

Why can screening be unhelpful? As I mentioned, the main reason we do screening tests is because we hope that by finding a disease earlier we could decrease suffering and prolong life or more generally, we do screening tests so that something useful can be done with the results. For that to happen the screening test has to be accurate, and the effective treatment has to be available. At present, neither is the case for prostate cancer screening. The test has many false-positives leading to unnecessary biopsies. Even when the test is right, the treatment does not seem to make much difference in survival while causing many side-effects (Coldman, 2003) (such as erectile dysfunction and urinary incontinence; which is true even for the so called nerve-sparing surgery). Nor does it seem to matter much whether or not your family member had prostate cancer (Makinen et al. 2002). It is for those reasons that The United States Preventive Services Task Force (the major organization providing evidence-based guidelines on prevention of illness) is stating that "the evidence is insufficient to recommend for or against routine screening for prostate cancer using prostate-specific antigen (PSA) testing or digital rectal examination (DRE)"[1] In this case, not only do we hurt many unnecessarily (by doing unnecessary biopsies and causing them to worry as a result of screening) but we are not even able to help the few who have the disease.

The value of screening mammography is questionable, though there is an appearance of uniform agreement. This issue has become political, which obscures objectivity. Screening mammography is a test that is far from perfect, and a woman has to be aware of the risks. First, there is a risk of false positive results. After ten years of screening, 23% of women who do not have cancer will have a false positive result and undergo additional procedures, 18% will undergo biopsies (Elmore et al., 1998). It is believed that breast cancer mortality is reduced in women age fifty-five to sixty-nine (Nyström et al., 2002), and possibly after age forty, (USPSTF,

---

[1] See http://www.ahrq.gov/clinic/3rduspstf/prostatescr/prostaterr.htm

2002) which is the currently recommended age of starting screening in the US. Some agencies recommend the extension of screening beyond age seventy-five (Randolph WM et al., 2002). Usefulness of screening mammography is probably higher in people with a family history of breast cancer (Kerlikowske et al., 1993).

Few agencies mention the risk of inducing breast cancer by mammography. A British agency (NHS Breast Screening Programme Publication No 54, 1997) calculated this risk for their screening population (women age 50-70). Lifetime risk varies with age; the younger you are at the time of first exposure, the higher the risk. This risk is additive: the more exposures you have the higher the risk. It is calculated that at age 60 *a single* two-view mammogram will cause cancer in 1:23000 women (based on the information and technology available in 1997). For a woman who follows US guidelines for screening, by age 65 a conservative estimate would be 1:1000 (one woman in one thousand would develop breast cancer as a result of radiation exposure from mammography). This is assuming that there were no false positives and additional mammographies were not performed. The British find that risk to their women (*who are screened from age 50 to 70 every 3 years with a two-view mammogram making it a total of six to seven mammograms*) is acceptable, because for every one cancer induced, 100 breast cancer deaths are possibly prevented. In the US we do a lot more screening than in the UK, consequently making this ratio less favorable.

I leave it up to each individual woman to decide whether this ratio is favorable enough for her. The United States Preventive Services Task Force quotes a 1997 review of risk estimates provided by the Biological Effects of Ionizing Radiation report of the National Academy of Sciences, estimating that annual mammography of 100,000 women for ten consecutive years beginning at age forty would result in up to eight radiation-induced breast cancer deaths. No woman would want to be one of those eight. To clarify, there is no discrepancy here in the numbers of women estimated to be affected by the radiation. The British state how many women would *get* cancer, the Americans state how many will *die* from cancer. The number is different because many women who will get breast cancer from screening mammography will die from something else, of old age for example.

In addition, strong evidence recently appeared questioning whether there is any mortality benefit from screening mammography at all (Cochrane Review on Screening for Breast Cancer with Mammography,

2001). European researchers analyzed the available data and found that while breast cancer related mortality is reduced, *total mortality is not*. This means that women whose cancers were detected by mammography died of something other than their cancer (perhaps of "natural" causes or from consequences of treatments, not reaping any of the benefit from the screening). They did not live longer than those whose cancers were never detected by screening mammography. This study is very controversial, but of good quality. More studies are under way. Another more recent study confirms the suspicion that mammography does no more than diagnose more cancers without a survival benefit (Sahl et al., 2004). This study of 4.3 million women in Sweden and Norway showed that with the introduction of mammography, there was a 54% increase in new diagnosis of invasive cancer among women between 50 and 69 years of age, but no decrease of new diagnosis of cancer among women older than 69. If cancer screening worked and we discovered and treated more cancers earlier, we should see a decrease of new cancers later, that's the point of screening. This study shows that this is not happening. That screening mammography leads to diagnosing more cancers, but nothing more. Some of these cancers that are now discovered would otherwise never have been found and never would have bothered those who had them.

To put this into simpler terms, before screening mammography was introduced, women were diagnosed with breast cancer when they came to the doctor with a big lump that they could no longer ignore. Mammography was supposed to allow detection of this lump much earlier so that by the time women were older fewer newly undiagnosed cancers would remain. In fact, the same number of women came to their doctor with a big lump after age sixty nine (screening was only done between ages fifty and sixty nine) as before mammography was introduced. The only difference was that many more women were labeled with having cancer, and given probably unnecessary treatment. This goes along with the other study that questions the usefulness of screening mammography. I do not know the main reason for being so attached to the idea of breast cancer screening. It may be our wish to believe that we can do something in a situation where we really can't, at least not so far. It may be the reluctance to acknowledge that what we've been doing for years has not been really helpful. It may be a fear that many jobs would be lost if screening mammography became a thing of the past. There surely are other reasons, but none is good enough to continue causing harm.

Another routinely performed screening test in pregnant women is a multiple marker screen or triple screen. It is a blood test to screen for Down's syndrome. Chances of having a baby with Down's syndrome vary with age a great deal, ranging from one in 1550 for women younger than twenty, to one in twenty-five for women older than forty-five years of age (Robbins Pathologic Basis of Disease, 2004). An authority called ACOG (American College of Obstetrics and Gynecology) recommends that *all* pregnant women under thirty five years of age be offered the test (ACOG Committee Opinion, 1994). Women over thirty-five are offered more aggressive invasive testing because of increased chances of them having a Down's syndrome baby (about one in 380 for a 35 year old woman). Follows is an example of is how this practice is affecting patients.

Patient/Family Perspective

An eighteen year old woman whom I saw for prenatal care became interested when I offered a multiple marker screening test. It was an unintended pregnancy for this young woman and even as she was coming to see me for prenatal care, she shared with me that she was considering an abortion. She went through about two weeks of agony until she finally decided to keep the baby. Now her pregnancy was at eighteen weeks of gestation and it was time to offer the test. I explained to the patient that in a young woman like herself, it was extremely unlikely that she would have a Down's baby. I also explained that the test is not always accurate; if abnormal (as is the case with all screening tests), it will require confirmatory tests. In addition, it is expensive—which didn't bother her because she had insurance.

She had the test, and it came back positive. As in prior similar situations, I ordered an ultrasound for dating. Most of the time this test is erroneously positive when the dating of the pregnancy is wrong, but this time the ultrasound confirmed that the dating was correct. I explained to the patient that now she had an option to go for invasive testing or to leave things as they were since the chances she had a Down's baby were still very low even with a positive test. The young woman wanted to go to the next step, and I set up an appointment with a specialist who would do an additional ultrasound, counsel her, and do the procedure that's called amniocentesis. In this procedure, under ultrasound guidance, a needle is placed through the abdominal wall into the woman's uterus and some of the fluid is aspirated. This fluid contains fetal cells that can be analyzed, and a definitive answer as to whether or not the baby has a Down's syndrome can be given.

As we tried to set up an appointment with the specialist, we discovered that the young woman had not renewed her insurance policy and was now uninsured. The specialist's office told us that the procedure costs $2600, and they wanted a half in advance. The young woman was in tears, telling us that she has only $300 and pleading with us to fix this somehow. My medical assistant, one of the most industrious people I've met, managed to contact the right people at the insurance company and reinstate the health insurance of this young lady within several days.

Physician's Perspective

While all this was happening, I decided to look up the actual numbers and calculate the risk of having a Down's syndrome baby for this young woman with a positive triple screen test. A statistical tool we have to help us in this estimate is called 'positive predictive value.' It is the likelihood that a positive screening test (a test that comes back as abnormal) will actually mean that there is a problem. The calculation is greatly dependent on the prevalence or on how frequently the problem is encountered (this is true for any screening test). The test's accuracy also goes into the calculation, since every screening test gives some false positive results. For this test the false positive rate is about 8% (Benn, 2003). Testing for a rare problem is more likely to lead to a false-positive result than testing for a frequent one. To my amazement, the positive predictive value for this young woman's test was less than one percent (or to be more precise, one in five hundred). This meant that of 500 women of her age who test positive, only one actually has a Down's syndrome baby. This was difficult to believe and I asked my former residency director to verify my result, which he did. The procedure that is offered after the test is both unpleasant and carries a risk of a miscarriage. One woman in 200 will miscarry as a result of amniocentesis (Antsaklis et al, 2000). Other less frequent risks are also involved.

To me this seems like a very lousy test. When used for a young woman, more than 99 percent of the time it causes unnecessary worry, physical discomfort, and a significant risk of miscarriage, not to mention an enormous waste of money. The specialist was honest with my patient. He told her of the one in 200 risk of a miscarriage, and gave her the ratio of one in 500 as her chances of having a Down's syndrome baby after a positive triple screen. Luckily she made the right choice by deciding not to undergo the amniocentesis. With this ratio, the screening test does not seem justified. Even for a thirty-five year old woman the likelihood that a positive screening test means there is actually a Down's syndrome baby is only 3%, or one in 33. With the risk of miscarriage from amniocentesis being 1 in 200, for every six Down's syndrome babies identified there will be one test-induced miscarriage. Even this doesn't sound like a good solution to me. In the meantime I decided arbitrarily not to offer the test to women younger than twenty-five as this seems clearly a bad idea causing much unnecessary worry, many unnecessary doctor-caused miscarriages, and a big waste of money. I can't help but think that it is a scheme for sending more business to the specialists. The young woman I described went on to deliver a healthy baby boy whom I had the privilege of delivering and examining myself.

Societal Perspective

The medical establishment is continuously suggesting to the public that screening tests are of great value. Even the so called non-profit organizations are promoting it. I say "so-called" because they still are after profits and can go about this quite aggressively. Here, for example, is an article from a newsletter published by one hospital in Fall 2004. A urologist wrote an article encouraging men to come for prostate cancer screening—a practice that has no proven value. It is an article that sounds like an infomercial with a fictional title. The quotes of the patient in this article are genuine and sincere but the patient may not be aware of the whole story. I changed and removed names to preserve privacy.

"Prostate Cancer: A Treatable Reality for Men.

"[…] Richard Couper of Burnsville was diagnosed with prostate cancer in 1999 and his urologist began monitoring his PSA (Prostate Specific Antigen) levels."

"[…] And today, prostate cancer is affecting countless families across the country. In fact, it is likely that every man may encounter some type of prostate problem in his lifetime. According to the American Cancer Society, 220,900 men in the United States will be diagnosed with prostate cancer this year. It is the most common form of cancer in men over age 50, and is the second leading cancer killer. Fortunately, with quality healthcare, it is also one of the most treatable cancers." (This paragraph makes you scared first and then gives a false hope of putting yourself into the hands of the "quality healthcare." In fact one need not be scared at all.

Most men who have prostate cancer will die of other causes without ever being bothered by it. Studies have shown that 50% of men at age 70 and 80% of men at age 90, who died of other reasons, have some degree of prostate cancer. The important point is that they die of something else without ever knowing that they have cancer (Hollander, 1998). To say that this is one of the most treatable cancers is also misleading. You can treat it all you want, but who needs a treatment that does not prolong life and causes side-effects?)

"Prostate cancer is best treated when caught early—nearly 60 percent of all prostate cancers are discovered while they are still confined to the prostate. The five-year survival rate for men diagnosed with prostate tumors at this stage is close to 100 percent." (What I would have to add here is that this is true whether or not there was any treatment. This cancer is indolent, meaning that it usually progresses very slowly. People who have a metastatic prostate cancer may have had it for many years. They have nothing to regret, had it been discovered earlier, they would have gone through years of treatment with its side-effects and worries, but without a significant benefit. As I mentioned earlier, there is no evidence that the current treatment prolongs life. Another idea that I often hear from patients relates to their inordinate belief in treatment. Patients say: "My friend had prostate cancer for ten years and treatment held it under control, then it got away and spread." Patients believe that treatment they receive "holds" cancer. The data suggest that treatment makes very minimal impact. Had the patient done nothing, the cancer would likely still be held locally for ten years and when the time came it would spread. Credit for holding cancer should go to the person's natural capacity to resist, not to the treatment. Effectiveness of cancer treatments will be discussed in more detail in the following chapter.)

"PSA screenings and watchful waiting.

PSA blood tests are known to detect prostate cancers at a very early stage. However, because not every case of prostate cancer requires treatment, opinions on early PSA screening are varied. While treatment may improve the condition of the cancer, it may also create side effects and undesirable lifestyle changes. As Dr. John Smith, radiation oncologist at Appletown Hospital, notes, "It's often hard for patients to accept the fact that they have cancer, and it might be best left untreated." (This hardship would have been avoided if no screening took place. This cancer is not only best left untreated, but even better, left undetected because it won't affect lifespan of the majority of men. As stated above, half of men at age seventy have some degree of prostate cancer but most die of something else. If they were all screened, they would have been labeled with the disease and treated with harmful treatments for something that would never have bothered them.)

"As a result, some doctors and patients choose to practice "watchful waiting," during which PSA levels are monitored until they reach a level that the patient and doctor agree warrants treatment. Today, however, "watchful waiting," has become a less popular practice, as more patients are opting to address their cancer upon diagnosis." (They are opting for early treatment because they are misled into thinking that it helps.)

"Charles Bronson, M.D., of Riverbank Urology, recommends that men 50 or older have an annual rectal exam and PSA test. "If there is a strong family history of prostate cancer, then it's important to keep an eye on it earlier," he says. "In those cases, we'll start the surveillance at age 40." (This will assure that Riverbank Urology has a steady stream of business.)

"Early prostate cancer may not present any symptoms and can only be found with regular prostate examinations. Do not let fear and anxieties keep you from having the tests that can often detect, or help rule out, prostate cancer." (I would say quite the opposite; the best evidence so far shows that this cancer is best left not found.)

"Treating prostate cancer
"Prostate cancer treatments range from curative to palliative. Curative treatments such as surgery and radiation therapy are aimed at eliminating cancer. Palliative treatments include hormonal therapy" (which, I would add, turns a man virtually sexless), "certain types of radiation, and chemotherapy, but are focused more on improving quality of life than curing."

"Sit down with your urologist and figure out which treatment is the right option for you," recommends Dr. Smith. "It's a tough decision, and that's why it's so important for the patient to be informed."

"Richard Couper and his urologist decided surgery was his best option. This was followed by a PSA test every 90 days. When Richard's PSA levels began to rise and his doctor recommended treatment, Richard was able to make an informed decision based on the research he had done. He chose to utilize Appletown Hospital's IMRT (intensity modulated radiation therapy) capabilities—a powerful technology that targets tumors precisely, minimizing damage to surrounding tissues." (Surgery, recurrence, then radiation therapy; not a great bargain for this patient but a great chance for the hospital to advertise its IMRT technology, the technology that has no proven lifesaving benefit in the treatment of prostate cancer.)

"IMRT wasn't available to Richard near his home in Burnsville, but because it was available at Appletown Hospital's Regional Cancer Care Services, Richard didn't have to leave the region to receive this innovative treatment. "The Appletown community is fortunate to have a cancer treatment team and technology that are world class, as well as an extraordinarily highly trained and experienced group of doctors," says Paul Blake, Ph.D., Director of Cancer Services at Appletown Hospital.

Six weeks into his IMRT treatment, Richard's PSA test showed a 40% decrease. It was his lowest PSA reading in three years. He's thrilled that his quest for quality information and treatment was successful. He's looking forward to years of good times with his family." (The patient is happy about the apparent success, a 40% decrease in PSA level. The information that he was not offered was that if he had no treatment at all, chances are he would live just as long but he and his family wouldn't have to go through the cancer scare, and he wouldn't have to get surgery and radiation. Again, currently there is no evidence that the available treatment of prostate cancer prolongs life.)

The reasons for this enthusiasm became clearer to me when I considered a financial briefing that I attended at one hospital. There was another Medicaid cut in our region which meant that more people would become uninsured. The financial officer explained that it meant more free service given by the hospital. This is because hospitals are obliged to take care of people presenting to the emergency room regardless of their ability to pay. Many patients who lost their insurance would make the local ER their care provider. How will the hospital pay for all this free service? The strategy was simple. The patients with "good" insurance would pay for it. How? By raising the rates the hospital charges for the services. The health insurance of the well-insured will compensate for the loss of revenue to the uninsured. The hospital is highly interested in attracting patients with good health insurance. The surest way to find such patients is by encouraging screening. Who else will come in for an unpleasant and potentially very costly procedure if not the people with good health insurance who want to get a full use out of it and are not aware of the harm that it can cause, nor of the cost?

A recent survey of five hundred adults shows just how much we have bought into the idea of cancer screening (Schwartz et al., 2004). These were men age fifty or older and women age forty or older who did not have cancer. Almost all women reported having had mammographies and Pap smears, 71% of men had prostate cancer screening, 47% had colon cancer screening. Thirty eight percent experienced false positive results from their screening tests, meaning that the test came back as positive requiring additional confirmatory tests that indicated that there was in fact no cancer. They called the experience "very scary" or "the scariest time of my life" but most of them reported that they were glad anyway that they had undergone the original testing. Even more interestingly 86% said they would get total body CT scan if it were available. Among them, 85% would prefer getting such a scan to receiving $1000 in cash. The editor summarizing the article says with some irony: "Consumers are clearly buying the fruits of our high tech manhunt for cancer." I agree.

With many screening tests, as in the case of prostate cancer screening and the triple screen of pregnant women, matters have got to the point where, without being aware of it, the medical establishment systematically misleads the public. I say 'without being aware' because very few are really aware. I, for example, was not aware of how useless and harmful the triple screen can be until I made the calculation myself. Most physicians including myself have no time to do such verifications on a regular basis. Instead, we tend to trust the authority of the organizations providing us with guidelines. The reasons for this willingness to trust is not only the lack of time for verification, but also the security which following the guidelines affords. As mentioned earlier, a doctor is relatively well protected in case of a lawsuit, if he followed the guidelines. This is true almost regardless of what the patient's outcome is. So together, fear and convenience drive doctors to try to impose the guidelines upon their patients, without verifying whether the recommendations are really good for those patients. This is why I think that patients would be better off taking the responsibility for their health into their own hands rather than delegating it to their doctor, and why I think that it is better for the patient not to undergo a screening test at all rather then undergoing one without understanding it.

Patient/Family Perspective

Patients need not feel oppressed by their doctor's opinion. Physicians need to respect a patient's personal preferences, even when they seem irrational, simply because every human being has the right to make choices about personal health care. This, taken with the fact that medicine cannot provide a perfect solution (a solution without additional suffering) for any illness, further increases the importance of patient self-determination. How many of us disable our kitchen smoke alarms? (I'm not encouraging this practice.) I have to admit that I am guilty of it. Those who do this are usually aware that smoke alarms may save lives, but we make a choice that may be viewed as irresponsible or unintelligent. We decide that we don't want to be inconvenienced multiple times because of a small chance that one time this may save our lives. I would argue that, as in the matters of personal safety, in the matters of personal health an individual has to have a choice, and no one has the right to judge this choice.

What I would recommend to the patient, as I recommend to my family, is not to accept at face value the multitude of the screening campaigns. When a doctor recommends a screening test, ask how accurate the test is (what are the chances of getting a false-positive result) and what would be the next step if the test comes back positive (abnormal). In screening there is *always* the next test. Then ask, if the next confirmatory test comes back positive again, what other tests would be involved? There are usually other tests to determine the extent of the disease. Ask what the treatment entails and how effective it is. Most doctors won't have enough time to explain all that. You can then try to find this information on your own. British and Canadian screening guidelines are much more reasonable than those in the US. One useful publication is *Evidence Based Medicine Journal* from the *British Medical Journal* publisher, available online at http://ebm.bmjjournals.com/. Also see the Canadian Task Force on Preventive Health Care at http://www.ctfphc.org/. (Go to Topics and then the Recommendations section).

I think the medical establishment in these countries is less influenced by big business.

To sum up, the probability that a positive screening test will mean that you have the disease (as opposed to a false positive result) depends on how likely you are to have the illness that's being screened for. Even though most screening tests are recommended for everyone, it is also well known that some people are at higher risk than others. If you are not sure whether or not to have the test, inquire if you'd be at a high or low risk. If you are at low risk, the usefulness of screening goes down. You may also consider asking your doctor whether he has had the test himself or plans to have it. If you notice that the doctor is hesitating or not giving you a straight wholehearted yes, it usually means that he is not confident in the need for that test. Then ask yourself whether you really want to know what you may conceivably find out, and whether you really want to be involved in all that a test entails. Do not proceed with a screening test if you are not prepared to go all the way and jump through all the hoops of the confirmatory tests, exploratory tests, and treatments. Don't feel bad refusing a test that you don't fully understand. Getting a test does not cure the problem nor does it guarantee future health. If you understand all the implications and still want the test, then by all means go ahead with it. I hope that the article that I placed above in its entirety would be an example of many similar promotional articles one finds in the popular and official-looking press. It is not much more than an infomercial, and as with all infomercials, exaggerations and distortions are common.

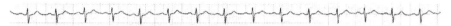

16 Illusions of Medical Omnipotence

Societal Perspective

I think that in medicine we often take credit for more than we deserve. We exaggerate our achievements, perhaps out of pride and as a reason to ask for more funding. Since we achieved this much, we obviously deserve more money so we can achieve more. While we made progress in some areas, other problems came to take their place. Sir William Osler (1849-1919) said "He who knows syphilis, knows medicine." He said this because in his pre-antibiotic era, treatment of syphilis was very complex, involving many side-effects, requiring treatment of the side-effects. Many people died and suffered severe complications. Today, once diagnosed in the early stages, it is very easy to treat, but other diseases have replaced it. In the 1980s one could say, "If you know AIDS you know medicine," because of a very similar situation we were in with AIDS. Progress seems to continue to march on, but one disease takes the place of another, and disease and death have not been conquered.

A Simple Example: Pharmacologic Omnipotence and the Search for the Perfect Drug

One can see a similar theme even in a disease like Parkinson's. Many advances and new medications have been invented, but all at a cost to the patient in terms of side-effects, and to the public in terms of money. Treatments are becoming more complex because they involve treatment of the side-effects. For example, a group of drugs for Parkinson's called 'dopamine agonists' can make one very sleepy, requiring the patient to take another drug to treat sleepiness. They also make one nauseous, requiring one to take an anti-nausea medication. Current treatments lose effectiveness with time, and new drugs are produced to improve efficacy. One other group of drugs called 'COMT inhibitors' are helpful, but also at a price of sleep attacks and liver toxicity. Yet another drug from a group called 'MAO-B inhibitors' causes a toxic interaction with some of the commonly used anti-depressants. Anti-parkinsonian drugs can cause hallucinations and delusions. To treat that, one needs to take an 'antipsychotic' drug that requires bi-weekly blood tests because it can cause serious blood abnormalities. Finally, in our age of advanced neurosurgery, a 'deep brain stimulation' device is available. It may sound like a great achievement until you learn that it only permits improvement of symptoms and reduction of the medication dosages for *several years* at the price of possible intracranial bleeding, partial paralysis and infection (Treatment Guidelines from The Medical Letter, 2004).

Drug recalls demonstrate another limitation of medicine. It takes time to discover whether a medication is really safe. A recent recall of Vioxx is but one of numerous examples. Before it was confirmed that it causes an increase in heart attacks and sudden cardiac death, (Topol & Falk, 2004) it got FDA approval for use in arthritis, migraines and menstrual pains. This is why, in spite of the fact that we are lead to believe in great importance of the latest breakthroughs, they rarely end up being as important as initially perceived.

Here is another example showing false excitement and urgency about the 'latest treatments.' I found this advertisement for a new cancer book on HealthNewsDigest.com. The book is entitled *Everyone's Guide to Cancer Therapy*. The excerpt says: "After receiving a diagnosis of terminal lung cancer in 1978, Bloch sought out a second opinion which proved lifesaving. After three years of successful treatment, Bloch came to the realization, "that if a doctor is unaware of the latest and best treatment for an individual patient, all the research—all the work done and all the money spent—is wasted as far as that patient is concerned. Many lives can be lost not because treatments to cure or control a cancer haven't been discovered, but because the physician may be unaware of them." The promoter here exaggerates quite a bit. It also sounds a lot like much of the healthcare advertising. It is aimed at creating a false sense of urgency, it is trying to say—"You better find the latest treatment or you will die!" The evidence says (as mentioned earlier in the book) that treatment of most lung cancers adds only a few months of life at best. This degree of life prolongation is not very impressive and it is not at all clear whether treatment is worth the trouble that the patient will have to go through.

A More Complex Example: Very Modest Effectiveness of Most Cancer Treatments

In my third year of medical school, which was not long ago (1999), an oncologist lecturing us said, "in spite of what you may have heard in the media, cancer, with the exception of childhood leukemias, testicular cancer, and Hodgkin's, is an incurable disease." This largely remains true today and has not changed much over the past decades. Fred Hutchinson Cancer Research Center lists the following cancers as being curable even after they have spread:

- Childhood Acute lymphoid leukemia (ALL)
- Hodgkin's disease
- Large cell lymphoma
- APL (acute promyelocytic leukemia)
- Testicular cancer
- Choriocarcinoma (rare cancer resulting from an abnormal pregnancy)

All other cancers are discussed in terms of survival (5, 10, 15 year survival). The cure is rare. Where do all the claims of cancer cure come from? A great deal of them, are from misleadingly equating pre-cancerous conditions with cancer. Many women who had some cellular changes of the breast tissue or on the cervix are led to believe that they had cancer and that it was cured. Terminology may be confusing here. In the breast these are called 'Ductal Carcinoma In Situ' (DCIS) or 'Lobular Carcinoma In Situ' (LCIS), on the cervix they are called 'Atypical Squamous Cells of Undetermined Significance' (ASCUS), 'Low/High Grade Squamous Intraepithelial Lesion' (LGSIL, HGSIL), or 'Cervical Intraepithelial Neoplasia' I, II, III (CIN-I, II, III). All these fancy terms have words in them that sound like cancer where in fact *they are not*. When curing these is counted as cancer cures, we seem very powerful. When you look at the facts our cures are a lot less impressive.

Let's start with a cervical cancer. Most of the changes in ASCUS and LGSIL, and 35% of HGSIL will return to normal spontaneously within 24 months (Melnikow et al, 1998). The treatment for HGSIL is either cryotherapy (freezing) or excision (with a knife or electricity). So, the majority of the women whom the medical system is treating and taking credit for, would have been fine without any treatment. While these preventive measures are effective in reducing the incidence of future cervical cancer, they are just that—preventive measures, not cures.

Breast cancer is a more dramatic example. It is estimated that about 20% of women will develop 'carcinoma in situ' (either lobular or ductal). The significance of this lesion is not known. Carcinoma in situ, although it sounds like cancer, is not a cancer at all. In cancer, abnormal cells grow beyond their boundaries and invade surrounding tissues. The words 'in situ' means that the abnormal cells have not gone beyond any boundaries (even microscopically). Lobules and ducts are the components of a breast. Lobular or ductal carcinoma in situ, are a collection of abnormal cells that is not growing beyond its microscopic boundaries. It is known that *most of them regress spontaneously*, without ever turning into cancer. It is also known that they are associated with cancer down the line, but what percentage will turn into cancer, what percentage will remain unchanged, and what percentage will regress spontaneously is not known. Studies indicate that approximately a third will develop into invasive cancer eventually (Ottesen, 2003), but all of them are treated, and credit is taken for all. With the advent of screening mammography, detection rates of these pre-cancerous conditions have been increasing. The two combined (DCIS and LCIS) now comprise 40% of newly diagnosed cancers (Abeloff, 2004). At least two thirds of those never would have bothered the women in whom they were detected. These are not cancers in spite of the word carcinoma in their name.

My suspicion about the cancer treatment hype was confirmed when I stumbled upon the article of Dr. Groopman in *The New Yorker* magazine and on a review of his recent book, "The Anatomy of Hope", in one of the professional newsletters (Groopman, 2001; Groopman, 2003). Dr. Jerome E. Groopman holds the Dina and Raphael Recanati Chair of Medicine at the Harvard Medical School and is Chief of Experimental Medicine at the Beth Israel Deaconess Medical Center. In his essay for *The New Yorker* magazine in 2001, entitled *The Thirty Years' War*, he gives a perspective of thirty years of cancer research.

Dr. Groopman mentions that a few weeks before he wrote his essay, *Barron's Magazine* had an article entitled "Investing in Health: Curing Cancer." The article ended by saying that "we are finally winning the war," and that for our children cancer will become just another chronic illness, for which they will only need to "pop a few pills every day."

Further, Dr Groopman describes how the optimism at the annual meeting of the American Society of Clinical Oncology, led to a surge of share prices of biotechnology and pharmaceutical companies. Political leaders were involved in planning funding and research in the new millennium. He says, that while there were some grounds for optimism, "…oncologists and cancer patients have been caught in a cycle of euphoria and despair as the prospect of new treatments has given way to their sober realities…"

A government-guided anti-cancer campaign was started by Mary Lasker, who was a prominent and influential cancer activist of the 60s and 70s. She persuaded the congress and President Nixon to pass the National Cancer Act, which was signed into law in December of 1971. The President would now appoint the director of the National Cancer Institute. Nixon declared, "This legislation—perhaps more than any legislation I have signed as President of the United States—can mean new hope and comfort in the years ahead for millions of people in this country and around the world..."

In the 1970s, no single chemotherapeutic agent was effective. One of the first effective combinations of chemotherapeutic drugs was developed by Dr. Vincent DeVita for a cancer called large-cell lymphoma. Numerous studies then followed to compare it to other known ineffective treatments. This resulted in a great deal of patient suffering and expenditure of millions of dollars.

Dr. Groopman described his grandmother's saga with a bone marrow cancer called chronic myelogenous leukemia. Her doctor told her that the scientists were close to identifying the virus that causes cancer. At that time, it was thought that viruses were primarily responsible for cancers. She was told that new and effective treatments would soon be available. That was in 1972. After undergoing many treatments that had numerous side-effects and have been since invalidated, she passed away in 1976.

In 1983, as a researcher, Dr. Groopman participated in a study of interferon for cancer. They were flooded with desperate requests from cancer patients wishing to participate in the study. As a typical example, he describes a patient, a middle-aged school teacher, who entered a study to treat melanoma. Again, after experiencing numerous side-effects of treatments, she died five months after enrolling in the study. Interferon was later found helpful in a rare cancer called hairy-cell leukemia, but it turned out to be ineffective in melanoma.

Dr. Groopman describes several patients with similar stories throughout the years of his career. New drugs were substituted for old ones, giving rise to new waves of enthusiasm followed by disappointments. He quotes the statistician John Bailar, who said: "In the nineteen-fifties, there was huge excitement about laboratory programs to screen for chemotherapy drugs...We found a few drugs, but not many. Then, in the nineteen-seventies, there were cancer viruses. In the eighties, it was immunotherapy, with biologics like interferon and interleukin-2 as the model magic bullets. Now it's cancer genetics. The rhetoric today sounds just the way it did forty years ago. I have no doubt that there has been a huge increase in knowledge about cancer. The problem is to translate it into public benefits we can measure. I want to see an impact on population mortality rates. If the treatments are really that good, then we'll see it."

Dr. Groopman also quotes Fran Visco, who is the president of the National Breast Cancer Coalition. She was dismayed at the way researchers interacted with members of the press. "These clinical scientists receive media training and are scripted by their hospitals…There are so many agendas here: fame, patient referrals, fund-raising, pharmaceutical grants, academic advancement." He also quotes Ellen Stovall, the president of the National Coalition for Cancer Survivorship, who agreed: "The headlines are dreadful." She referred to the sensationalism surrounding the disease as "the pornography of cancer," adding, "I am excited by the new science, but show me hard data. We need to raise the skepticism barometer."

Looking at a more recent article in *The Economist* magazine, one can see that story we are told is not changing. Now, in 2004, the cover page of the October 16th issue reads: ***Beating cancer.*** Now for the thirty-third year in a row, we continue to be on a verge of a major breakthrough. One can also learn here about the amounts of money being spent. As one can see, it appears to present very good news—beating cancer. The introduction is cheerful: "After long years of disappointment in the war against cancer, a new front is opening up. There may never be a cure, but new methods and better treatments will make the many diseases which go by that name far less scary." One could easily fall for these promises, if one was unaware that there had been many promises made and not kept. This was shown in the essay by Dr. Groopman, and, I hope, will be seen with greater clarity in my review of the currently available data below.

If you read more, the news becomes more realistic (The Economist., Oct 16, 2004): "Going by the numbers, humanity seems to be losing the war on cancer. According to the most recent data from the World Health Organisation, 10 m[illion] people around the planet were diagnosed with the disease in 2000, and 6 m[illion] died from it. And these numbers are growing. With an ageing population, the spread of western-style diets, and increasing tobacco consumption, cancer is on the rise around the globe. In America, for example, projections suggest that 40% of those alive today will be diagnosed with some form of cancer at some point in their lives. By 2010, that number will have climbed to 50%."

"All this is despite the fact that, since then-president Richard Nixon's famous speech in 1971, launching what became known as the war on cancer, America has given nearly $70 billion (in actual, not inflation-adjusted, dollars) to its National Cancer Institute (NCI). And that is not to mention the money spent by drug companies and charities—nor, indeed, the research budgets of other countries. Despite these billions, the rate of death from cancer in the United States has increased from 163 per 100,000 individuals in 1971 to 194 per 100,000 in 2001."

The article ends on an optimistic note with little evidence to support this optimism: "Luckily, these numbers do not tell the whole story. In fact, scientists are optimistic about the future of cancer treatment. Very optimistic. As Paul Workman, director of the Cancer Research UK Centre for Cancer Therapeutics, a charity, puts it, 'This is the second golden era of cancer research.' While no one expects a cure for cancer in the next decade, many think it could be demoted to the status of a chronic disease that people can live with—in other words, something more like diabetes."

I hope Mr. Workman is right, but I wouldn't hold my breath. The scientists are usually optimistic when their livelihood depends on this optimism.

This unwarranted optimism leads the public to have false beliefs of medical omnipotence. Dr. Kopes-Kerr, in a review of Dr. Groopman's book in his professional newsletter, cites him calling the cancer establishment, *"that immense whirligig of doctors, scientists and pharma-companies, [which] had systematically misrepresented the prospect of hope to millions of patients."* Dr. Kopes-Kerr comments to his readers, "Screening, cancer detection, and cancer treatment are inextricably intertwined. Are we selling lies or realistic hope and can we tell the difference? Hard to know but worth thinking about." (Kopes-Kerr, 2004)

Cancer related issues involve a great deal of suffering, fear, and money. "Cancer is the second leading cause of death in the United States and is expected to become the leading cause of death within the next decade." (Stewart SL, et al., 2004) According to American Cancer Society estimates, cancer caused approximately 556,000 deaths in 2003. (Kumar: Robbins and Cotran: 2005) Below is a table (Table 16-1.) of deaths from the most common cancers. (Data for 2000 is from Noble: Textbook of Primary Care Medicine, 3rd edition. For 2003 estimates from: Abeloff: Clinical Oncology, 3rd ed., 2004 Elsevier, U.S. Cancer Burden 2003 estimates of expected new cases and deaths in relation to other organ sites.)

Type of cancer	Deaths in 2000	Deaths in 2003
Lung	156,900	157,200
Breast	41,200	39,800
Colon	56,300	57,100
Prostate	31,900	28,900

**Table 16-1: Number of Deaths From
the Most Common Cancers in 2000 and 2003**

These figures are usually presented to support the need for more research and funding. With time, however, they also begin to convey a lack of effectiveness of our methods. They represent much unnecessary suffering, many false hopes, and many billions of dollars spent.

Trying to figure out **how much benefit one can expect from treating cancer** is complicated. On the one hand, we hear constant claims of success and improved survival, on the other hand there are reports showing very minimal changes over the past forty years.

Lung cancer is the leading cause of cancer death in both men and women in the United States and accounts for 28% of all cancer deaths. (Murray & Nadel, 2000). Therefore, I started my search with lung cancer. My aim was to find out how much benefit one can gain from treating this cancer with all of the modern medical treatments. What kind of information do we usually see when we try to find out about effectiveness of a certain treatment? One of the usual ways is to look at the systematic reviews of the effectiveness of certain treatments. These are well established, standardized scientific methods of reviewing data. Here is an example of one such report of effectiveness of certain chemotherapeutic agents on 'Non-Small Cell Lung Cancer', which is the most common group of lung cancers:

> Median survival was improved with docetaxel compared to best standard care (75 mg/m2 gave an extra 3 months' survival). No difference in median survival was shown between docetaxel and vinorelbine or ifosamide... paclitaxel improved survival by 2 months compared to best standard care. Comparisons with other drugs showed mixed results and no clear survival advantage. Only one trial showed a worsening effect on quality of life with paclitaxel-cisplatin at 12 weeks (but not

at 6 weeks) compared to cisplatin-teniposide. Other comparisons showed little difference.

No difference in survival was shown in three trials of gemcitabine verus older drugs, while two trials showed an improvement of about 6 weeks. Compared to best standard care, no difference was shown in survival but quality of life was improved. Quality of life was not improved with gemcitabine compared to older drugs. (Clegg A, 2001)

This is quite typical. Some drugs increased survival by two months, others by three, yet others did not help at all. One tends to think that these increments of two to three months have added up to something more substantial over the past forty years. The first chemotherapeutic agents, most of which are now obsolete, came out about forty years ago. In fact, the process is more complicated than simply adding things up.

The factors that influence survival include the destructive effects of the medications used. Chemotherapy tries to kill the cancer before killing the patient, but it doesn't always work out that way. Estimates of survival are influenced by how early the cancer is detected. Detecting cancer earlier in its course, as is done with screening, may create an impression of prolonged survival. This is called 'screening effect.' Another factor is finding cancers that would never bother the person who has them. That happens when an early stage cancer is discovered in an old person. Besides these contributors to apparent cancer survival, there is an important contributor to a decrease in cancer mortality that has nothing to do with treatment. It is the effect of preventive measures and general health promotion. Smoking cessation results in a decline of lung cancer mortality. Detection of precancerous conditions by a Pap smear, with subsequent treatment, results in a decline of cervical cancer mortality. Again, doing Pap smear too frequently can also be harmful. Balance needs to be reached. The preventive measures are enormously helpful, but have nothing to do with the cancer treatment.

Few placebo-controlled studies are now performed on cancer patients. Much more commonly, the old regimens are compared to the new ones. Here is an example of a review that tried to compare survival of patients with extensive 'Small Cell Lung Cancer' (SCLC), who were given chemotherapy, with those who were given placebo, "Ifosfamide gave an extra 78.5 days survival (mean survival time) compared with the placebo group. Partial tumour response was greater with the active treatment. Toxicity was only seen in the chemotherapy group. Pooled analysis was not possible because only mean survival time was reported in both studies for patients with extensive disease." Reviewers' conclusions: "Chemotherapeutic treatment prolongs survival in comparison with placebo in patients with advanced SCLC. Nevertheless, the impact of chemotherapy on quality of life and in patients with poor prognosis is unknown." (Agra, 2003) Here, with extensive lung cancer, the reviewer concludes that seventy eight days is a significant increase in survival, admitting that it comes at the cost of toxicity. Not many patients, however, would agree that it is significant enough for them, if they knew all that the treatment entails.

One good way of evaluating the benefit of cancer treatment is by comparing what is called *relative cancer survival.* "Relative survival compares the observed survival for a group of cancer patients with the survival of members of the general population who have the same characteristics, such as, age, gender, and [place] of residence, as the cancer patients. For example, women with a relative survival from breast cancer of 80% are 80% as likely to live another 5 years as are women of the same age who live in the same province." (Canadian Cancer Society, 1992) Below is a table (Table 16-2.) showing the figures of relative cancer survival in lung cancer by year of diagnosis, race and gender (Data from Ries et al, 1998.).

YEAR OF DIAGNOSIS	MEN		WOMEN	
	White	Black	White	Black
1960-1963	7.0	5.0	11.0	6.0
1974-1976	11.1	11.0	16.0	13.1
1989-1994	13.0	9.7	16.5	13.9

Table 16-2: Five-Year Relative Cancer Survival for Lung Cancer by Year of Diagnosis, Race and Gender

You may note that while survival doubles in relative terms (from seven to thirteen in white men), in absolute terms, a change from seven to thirteen percent is not as impressive. You may also note that almost all of the increase occurred between 1960s and 1970s with almost no increase since then.

The picture becomes more complicated with cancers that we screen for, namely breast, prostate, and colon cancer. Here, screening results in detection of earlier stages of cancer. In addition to possibly making such cancers easier to treat, this also creates an appearance of longer survival regardless of treatment. To put it in more simple terms, when a man develops a large tumor in his prostate at eighty years of age, one year before he dies, his survival is one year. Now we can detect the same cancer ten years earlier by a screening test. The man gets treated for eleven years and still dies at eighty one. His survival now is reported to be eleven years. This is how the impact of screening may appear far more effective than it actually is.

There is no secret, in the scientific medical circles, that the issue of effectiveness of treatment is not settled. Here is an example of a conclusion from a study done in Spain in year 2000. "Today, the use of PSA (a screening test for prostate cancer) allows doctors to diagnose prostate cancer at earlier stages and in younger patients. This has lead to an increase in the frequency of radical prostatectomy (a major prostate surgery with multiple side-effects). Future research should investigate whether this increase in radical prostatectomy has significantly changed the mortality rate of patients with prostate cancer." (Mesa, 2000) Note that the increase in prostate surgeries had started before there were any data to show that the surgery prolongs life. Such is usually the case. When we find something wrong, we want to do something about it, even before we know whether our intervention will help or harm.

Here is an example of a study whose authors are optimists, believers in the usefulness of the PSA screening for prostate cancer:

> SEER data on prostate cancer incidence from 1988 through 1998 were consistent with overdiagnosis rates of approximately 29% for whites and 44% for blacks among men with prostate cancers detected by PSA screening. Conclusions: Among men with prostate cancer that would be detected only at autopsy, these rates correspond to overdiagnosis rates of, at most, 15% in whites and 37% in blacks. The observed trends in prostate cancer incidence are consistent with considerable overdiagnosis among PSA-detected cases. However, the results suggest that the majority of screen-detected cancers diagnosed between 1988 and 1998 would have presented clinically and that only a minority of cases found at autopsy would have been detected by PSA testing. (Etzioni, 2002)

The authors here try to justify screening, by saying that only the minority of the discovered cancers would not ever have bothered the patients in whom they were found. Even with their conservative estimates, this constitutes 15% of whites and 37% of blacks screened in the US. Of note here, also, is the usual fact that whenever there is suffering—the minorities suffer more.

An even more recent study from the Wayne State University School of Medicine and the Barbara Ann Karmanos Cancer Institute in Detroit, Michigan came up with the following conclusion when looking at the metastatic prostate cancer survival changes from 1973 to 1997: "Relative survival has increased over the past three decades although this trend is **not statistically significant** [emphasis added]." (Barnholtz-Sloan, 2003) Remember, the seventy-eight day increase in survival in lung cancer, in the studies mentioned earlier, was considered statistically significant. Well, this finding isn't even statistically significant. The standard scientific methodology calls for disregarding of any trends or results that are not statistically significant.

With the following examples of breast cancer survival information, I hope to illustrate further nuances that affect our perception of effectiveness of treatment. In the table below (Table 16-3.) you can see the kind of information most doctors look at, and give to their patients. (Data adapted from Abeloff: Clinical Oncology, 3rd ed., Copyright © 2004 Elsevier, which adapted the data from Early Breast Cancer Trialists' Collaborative Group: Systemic treatment of early breast cancer by hormonal, cytotoxic, or immune therapy: 3 randomized trials involving 31,000 recurrences and 24,000 deaths among 75,000 women. Lancet 992;339:1)

10-Year Risk of Death From Breast Cancer	Example Of Patients With Early Breast Cancer At Such Risk
10–20	Stage I, good prognosis
20–40	Stage I, poor prognosis
40–80	Stage II, any prognosis

Table 16-3: Risk of Death From Breast Cancer

Ten year risk of death from breast cancer in Table 16-3 is a relative or *cancer-specific risk*. The significance of this will become clearer by exploring the data in Table 16-4. (Table created from the data adapted from Sutherland, 1986)

Years of Survival	5	10	15	20	30
Survival from All Causes or Total Survival	62%	43%	33%	25%	18%
Breast-cancer specific Survival	76%	65%	63%	61%	59%

Table 16-4: Comparison of Total Survival with Cancer-Specific Survival in Stage III-IV Breast Cancer

The data here come from patients with stage III-IV breast cancer. In this table, I placed the data of total survival next to the data on cancer-specific survival to demonstrate the difference between the two. The cancer-specific survival (or breast cancer-specific survival) is always greater. The doctor will usually tell you (looking at this table) that you have a 65% chance of surviving your breast cancer after ten years. What the patient *really* needs to know is *total survival*. Cancer-specific survival does not take into account other causes of death that a cancer patient will face. Comparing cancer-specific survival with healthy persons' survival leads to overestimation of the effect of treatment. While cancer-specific mortality may decrease as a result of treatment, total mortality may not, as seen in the data presented earlier on breast cancer. In simpler terms, a woman treated with chemotherapy for her breast cancer becomes immuno-suppressed as a result of chemotherapy. She then develops pneumonia and dies. In the statistics she will be counted as a triumph of modern medicine—she did not die of breast cancer. A study that does not look at total mortality will look at one hundred of such women and say—"our interventions decreased *breast cancer deaths* (or cancer-specific mortality), we should continue intervening." Beware when you hear of decreasing breast cancer deaths, prostate cancer deaths or other cancer deaths. These terms mean cancer specific survival and do not reveal whether treatment makes one live longer. It is an unfortunate and misleading artifact of modern medical terminology.

I am far from being the first one to look into the effectiveness of cancer treatment. One study published in the year 2000 looked at the increases of survival comparing them to decreases in mortality. If increase in survival is due to effective treatment we should see a decrease in mortality. Researchers looked at the twenty most common tumors. "From

1950 to 1995, there was an increase in 5-year survival for each of the 20 tumor types. The absolute increase in 5-year survival ranged from 3% (pancreatic cancer) to 50% (prostate cancer). During the same period, mortality rates declined for 12 types of cancer and increased for the remaining 8 types. There was little correlation between the change in 5-year survival for a specific tumor and the change in tumor-related mortality. (This means that the cancers with improved survival did not show a concomitant decrease in mortality, indicating that it is not a true increase in survival.) On the other hand, the change in 5-year survival was positively correlated with the change in the tumor incidence rate. (It means that cancers were detected earlier by testing, creating an appearance of increased survival.) Conclusion: Although 5-year survival is a valid measure for comparing cancer therapies in a randomized trial, our analysis shows that changes in 5-year survival over time bear little relationship to changes in cancer mortality. Instead, they appear primarily related to changing patterns of diagnosis" (Welch HG, 2000). I described the exact same situation earlier, in the example of a man with prostate cancer. Here researchers found it to be true for a number of cancers. The pattern of diagnosis changes by the introduction of a screening test. Cancer is discovered earlier, and there is an appearance of longer survival. The patient gets treated and still dies close to the time when he would have died without any treatment. Sometimes the patient dies from other causes creating a decrease in cancer specific mortality. The bottom line is that total mortality has improved only for a few rare cancers.

The National Cancer Institute collects data on 5-year relative cancer survival, and makes it publicly available[1]. The data in table 16-5 are adapted from this source. (SEER Program, NCI, based on an approximate 10 percent sample of the U.S. population.)

Here you can see for yourself the degree of improvement from 1974 to 1990. Not all of the modest increases in survival are attributable to treatment. As described above, some of it is due to early detection. Analysts of the data at NCI confirm this: "The overall 5-year relative survival rate for all cancer sites combined increased slightly from 49.3 percent in 1974-76 to 53.9 percent in 1983-90. Early data from 1960-63 and 1970-73 were not available for all races combined. Survival rates vary by primary site from less than 3 percent for cancer of the pancreas to more than 90 percent for cancer of the thyroid.

---

[1] See http://seer.cancer.gov/publications/

Type of Cancer	5-year relative survival in 1974-1976	5-year relative survival in 1983-1990
Lung	12.3%	13.4%
Breast	74.3%	80.4%
Prostate	66.7%	79.6%
Colon	49.5%	59.2%
All cancers combined	49.3%	53.9%

**Table 16-5: Five-Year Relative Cancer Survival Change
from 1974-1976 to 1983-1990**

Part of the recent increase in breast cancer survival may be due to early detection; a higher percentage of the more recent cases were diagnosed with smaller tumors. *Survival increases for prostate cancer may also in part be the result of early detection and the inclusion of occult disease in asymptomatic men."* (My emphasis).

Comparable data can be found in other countries. The Canadian Cancer Society[2] reports the following 5-year relative survival in 1992: "Five-year relative survival rates for ages 15–99 were highest for prostate cancer (87%), followed by breast cancer (82%), colorectal cancer (56% among men and 59% among women), and lung cancer (14% among men and 17% among women)."

Similar observations were made in Switzerland:

> This analysis with data from the cancer registry of the Saarland deals with 9 tumor localizations: stomach, colon, rectum; breast, cervix uteri and corpus uteri; prostate, lung, malignant skin melanoma. In general the 5-year relative survival rates slightly increased when the time period 1972-1976 was compared with 1982-1986. Cancer of the corpus uteri was one exception, in that the relative survival rate was constant over time, and cancer of the cervix uteri was another, in that a

---

[2] See http://www.cancer.ca/ccs/internet/standard/0,3182,3172_367655_39066503_langId-en,00.html

decrease of relative survival rate was found, which together with the decreasing incidence might be ascribed to a successful early detection program. There was no significant improvement in the relative survival time for lung or breast cancer patients. (Wiebelt, 1991).

This next article looked at the trends in cancer mortality in the US since 1990, and found decreases in mortality from breast and prostate cancer:

Statistically significant decreases in mortality among all races combined occurred with lung and bronchus cancer among men (-1.7%/year); colorectal cancer among men and women (-2.0%/year and -1.7%/year, respectively); prostate cancer (-2.6%/year); and female breast cancer (-2.3%/year). For 1990-2000, cancer mortality remained stable among American Indian/Alaskan Native populations. Statistically significant increases in lung and bronchus cancer mortality occurred among women of all racial/ethnic backgrounds, except among Asian/Pacific Islanders. Interpretation: Although cancer remains the second leading cause of death in the United States, the overall declining trend in cancer mortality demonstrates considerable progress in cancer prevention, early detection, and treatment. (Stewart, 2004)

As we can see, the greatest decreases in mortality are observed in breast and prostate cancer, followed by colon cancer. These are the three cancers affected by the screening effect. While it is possible that cancer mortality truly decreases, one needs to note that there may be several explanations for that. As mentioned in the quote, prevention accounts for some of the decrease (i.e. quitting smoking prevents lung cancer). Another aspect not accounted for is that cancer-specific mortality and total mortality aren't the same thing. Do treated patients live longer because of the treatment? The currently available data say that, if there is such a benefit, it is very small, except with a few rare cancers.

Other Examples

The statistical tools used to present the data influence the way we perceive it. This misperception backfired in the case of hormone replacement therapy. When the adverse effects of hormone replacement therapy were discovered, the relative risks were presented to the public and to the physicians. The relative risks always appear dramatic, but what we really need to know is the absolute risk, or the actual numbers. With hormone replacement therapy, the relative risk of breast cancer is increased by 26% which sounds like a lot (Grimes & Lobo, 2002). The absolute risk (the actual numbers) is an increase of breast cancer incidence from 30 per 10,000 in women not taking HRT to 38 in 10,000 in those taking it (Abeloff: Clinical Oncology, 3rd ed., 2004). This sounds a lot less dramatic, though it represents exactly the same data. After looking at the absolute risk numbers, one would not panic, there is a small increase in cancer, but it is very small. Here this statistical trick was used to create big headlines, but it is more commonly used in inflating the perception of effectiveness of a medication.

One of the professional newsletters provides an excellent example, "ads tout a 67% lower risk of patients stopping *Biaxin XL* compared to regular *Biaxin* due to side effects. This sounds dramatic...but it really isn't. The 67% is a RELATIVE risk reduction. The ABSOLUTE risk reduction is only 2%...a difference from 3% to 1% of all patients." (Prescriber's Letter, 2004) In other words, instead of 3% of patients who discontinued the drug due to side-effects, 1% discontinued with a new formulation. This is an improvement, but a very modest one. But the statistical tools allow one to claim a relative risk reduction of 67%, which sounds very dramatic.

Another less dramatic but still interesting source of information comes from a recent movement in medicine called 'evidence-based medicine'. Tools were invented to have a practical idea of how useful many of the commonly used treatments are. One way to express this is 'Number Needed to Treat' (NNT). I think many would find it surprising to learn that the treatments we use for many common illnesses make no difference for the majority of patients taking them. NNT is the number that expresses how many patients need to be treated for a certain condition in order to see a benefit from the treatment in one patient. Similarly 'Number Needed to Harm' (NNH) is the number of patients that need to be treated before we will see a harmful effect of therapy in one patient. Here is a list of some of these (Prescriber's Letter, Oct. 2004).

For the new guideline of lowering LDL, (the bad) cholesterol, down to 70 in very high risk patients, the NNT is 50, meaning fifty patients have to be treated for one year to lower their LDL cholesterol to 70 as opposed to 100, in order to prevent one heart attack. This ratio is not too bad but surely shatters the idea that everyone taking the medication is prevented from getting a heart attack. Over the course of ten years, this ratio may presumably rise to one in five. That's a long time with a lot of pills, blood tests, and side effects to prevent one heart attack in five people.

For mild hypertension (systolic blood pressure up to 160, diastolic up to 100) the NNT is 700, meaning 700 people need to be treated for one year to prevent one stroke, heart attack, or death. So you might estimate that after taking pills daily for ten years the chances that it would help you is only 1 in 70, and in 20 years, only 1 in 35. It is nice that it helps but would it be worth the inconvenience of taking the pill every day for twenty years and getting occasional side-effects? I don't think that every patient would agree.

With severe hypertension, the odds of getting a benefit are much better, the NNT is 15; so if fifteen patients take a pill for one year, one stroke, heart attack, or death will be avoided.

With hormone replacement therapy, you get the following trade-off: 333 patients need to be treated for five years to prevent one hip fracture and one colorectal cancer. On the other hand, after 250 people take it for five years, one will get a stroke, one will get a heart attack (Number Needed to Harm is 250 for those), one in 200 will get a breast cancer, and one in 100 will get a blood clot in the deep veins of the leg.

For ear infection in children more than 2 years of age, the NNT is 15, meaning that fifteen children need to be treated to relieve pain in one; for younger children the number is 9. The NNH is 12, meaning that after treating twelve kids, one will get a side-effect such as a rash, vomiting, or diarrhea.

For prevention of infection after a dog bite, sixteen need to take an antibiotic to prevent one infection.

For influenza, twenty-three persons need to get a vaccine to prevent one case of influenza.

For strep throat, 3000-4000 people need to be treated to prevent one case of acute rheumatic fever (which is the only important reason we treat strep throat).

In stroke prevention, when attempting to prevent a first stroke, sixty-seven people have to take aspirin for one year to prevent one stroke. To prevent a subsequent stroke, forty people have to take aspirin for one year to prevent one stroke.

In dementia, eight patients have to take Gingko for one year for one to have a 4 point improvement on a cognitive scale.

For prevention of hip fractures in the elderly, fourteen have to take Calcium 1200 mg with vitamin D for three years to prevent any fracture, twenty to forty to prevent a hip fracture. This is pretty good considering that this product is cheap, without significant known side-effects, and with lots of other benefits.

Patient/Family Perspective

Conclusion: What Should a Patient with Cancer Do?

What would I recommend to a person who is seeking treatment for cancer? Find out exactly what the treatment is going to bring you in terms of prolongation of life and quality of life. Find out what the treatment is going to involve, what side-effects, time commitments, frequency of visits for follow-ups, frequency of blood tests, chances of having to be hospitalized for treatment of the side-effects. Proceed when you understand the answers and the uncertainties involved and it still seems worthwhile. If it does not seem worthwhile, do not waste your time and resources on it. Seek alternative treatments and ask the same questions plus estimate the expenses. A family member can help find answers but should not try to convince the patient. Family members can state their opinions when asked, but need to let the patient make up his or her own mind. No one can truly know the right answer, but we can know the answer that the patient prefers to go with. Finally, if one is dying, as Dr. Kopes-Kerr said about his own possibility of dying from colon cancer: "[Colon cancer] is a perfectly respectable cancer." This means that there is nothing wrong with dying of cancer. After all, it is the second leading cause of death in the US. When treatment does not seem to be helpful, one should not hesitate to refuse it. Comfort measures can always be undertaken without cancer treatments (chemotherapy, radiation, curative surgery). Do not lose hope. Though infrequent, there are multiple well documented cases of spontaneous remission from a variety of cancers including lung, breast, colon and prostate cancer, leukemia, lymphoma and many others (National Cancer Institute Monograph 44, Nov. 1976). In fact, even scientific research has found that *active coping style* (Faller, 2002) and *hopefulness* (Molassiotis et al, 1997) are associated with better survival in cancer patients. As Dr. Bernie Siegal says in his book *Love, Medicine, and Miracles*, "The only false hope is no hope." (Siegal, 1986)

Regarding other diseases, the 'Number Needed to Treat' figures that I presented above give some perspective. Most conditions are healed by themselves and our bodies and minds, not the medicines. Medications can be very helpful in many acute conditions, but for chronic diseases their effect is modest and often comes at a significant price—side effects.

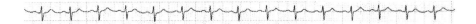

17 Patient Expectations and the Standard of Care

Physician's Perspective

In a recent study on evaluation of clavicular fractures (broken collar bones), physicians did very well diagnosing the problem, but sent everyone to get an X-ray anyway, even those patients in whom they had no doubt of the diagnosis (about a third of patients). The reasons they gave for sending patients for an unnecessary X-ray were *patient expectations* and "*standard of care*" (Shuster et al., 2004).

We discussed standard of care previously when describing the medical model and dealing with practice guidelines. The standard of care also involves local standards of care or what one may call a 'community standard.' These are the ways that things are done locally and are not always scientifically based. It is what is done in a particular hospital or region simply because of a habit. A physician asks himself *what will my colleagues think if I don't do what is customary to do here? Will they consider me a poor physician?* A good physician has to overcome this approval seeking.

Patient/Family Perspective

Suppose you are a patient and don't understand why something is being done. You can find out if the reason is merely compliance with a standard of care by asking for the reason. If the action is justified by referring to an extremely unlikely danger, you are probably dealing with a physician trying to fulfill a standard.

Physician's Perspective

In an outpatient setting this happens a lot with children. Standards from the American Academy of Family Practice and from the American Academy of Pediatrics say that they have to be checked for anemia around one year of age (American Academy of Family Physicians, 1999). This standard is not even universally agreed upon because other agencies debate its usefulness, (USPSTF, 1996) citing that there is insufficient evidence for screening infants who are not in high risk groups. Again you have to know what group you and your child belong to. If the child ends up having anemia, we'll give him multivitamins with iron and possibly do lead testing. The vitamin will almost always take care of the problem. Getting blood from an infant can be quite a struggle, but many physicians chose to put every child through it, just to comply with a standard. I think that if the child lives in a healthy environment, it is enough to ask a parent whether they think he needs a vitamin (if the child is a poor eater) and just give it to them, reserving blood testing for those who live in poor conditions.

Societal Perspective

While acting in accordance with a standard makes a doctor feel protected, the reverse is also true. A doctor who is not complying with a standard feels exposed to risk. After all, if something should go wrong and a lawyer reviews his chart, the doctor may appear incompetent. This drives many doctors to practice defensive medicine. All the tests that could possibly be done are done. With most tests, the normal values are established by testing healthy people and selecting the 95% closest to the mean to be the norm. That automatically puts five percent of healthy people outside the norm and subject to additional testing to confirm or refute the initial abnormal result. The patient is lucky if all the results are normal, but if not, he is destined to jump through the hoops like a lab animal. The result is both physical and emotional distress, and huge amounts of wasted money.

Physician's Perspective

Some community standards aren't even based on scientific evidence but rather on a habit. Thus in one of the hospitals where I work, if a patient comes in with a stroke and a neurologist is consulted, the patient will always get both aspirin and intravenous heparin. This is in spite of the fact that the neurologist's own authority—the American Academy of Neurology—recommends not to give intravenous heparin because a review of evidence shows that it causes increased risk of major bleeding and death without improving strokes (Coull et al, 2002). I suppose it is simply inertia—"we'll do it that way because we've done it that way for thirty years."

Recently this happened to one of the patients in my practice. My practice associate consulted a neurologist for a stroke patient he admitted. A neurologist initiated intravenous heparin infusion, which led to a major bleeding requiring a blood transfusion and a prolonged hospital stay.

Now, when I admit a patient with stroke, I am reluctant to consult a neurologist even when I need one. If you are in a similar situation, offered a treatment that has potentially serious harm, *ask how much benefit the treatment is likely to provide.* Then ask what about the likelihood of the adverse outcome. Then decide for yourself. If the doctor who offers you the treatment cannot give you the likelihood of benefit, it is best not to proceed with the treatment. That doctor may simply be following an old habit, a habit that is not based on any evidence.

Patient expectations invoke several mechanisms that also shape a great deal of what happens with medical diagnosis and treatment. One is fear of litigation; another is fear of appearing incompetent and losing a patient; yet another is optimizing the placebo effect, which is part of the art of medicine.

Societal Perspective

Linda Crawford, to whom I referred earlier in the book (Tracy, 2003), who teaches medical malpractice law at the Harvard Law School, says: "It is clear to us, 22 years into this research, that lawsuits are not about bad outcomes. They are not about bad relationships. They are about expectations."

"When we talk to our patients about treatment and operations, we do so through informed consent; yet, 31% of our malpractice cases at Harvard still have informed consent as a major component of the lawsuit. The basis of a patient's claim [might be] that they didn't understand that a complication was possible or that a certain outcome was possible after the operation. The physicians then say, very justifiably, "Look at it; you signed on the dotted line. This was a potential complication." But our actions speak louder than our words. Even for major invasive procedures, people don't even have to show up until the morning of the surgery. Often, as we go to surgicenters or as we go to day surgery, people have increasingly significant surgery where they don't even stay overnight. Furthermore, even if you have had major invasive surgery, you are out the door in a couple of days."

"What does that do for our patients? They say, 'Well, how serious can this be?' And in that regard, we are the victims of our own success when it comes to medical malpractice lawsuits. People's expectations rise. [They assume that the surgery] can't be all that serious, or they'd be keeping them in the hospital for a few days. When you actually do have a surgical complication, even a well-known surgical complication, you have a gap in expectations. What saddens me, as somebody who spends a great deal of time with physicians who are going through malpractice lawsuits and knowing how destructive the legal system is to good physicians, is that the more medical advances we make, the higher the expectations. And the higher the expectations, the greater the number of lawsuits regardless of the quality of our medicine."

Most physicians are aware of this and will be very reluctant to take a course of action that is contrary to patient expectation. If the patient expects getting an X-ray, few will refuse and fewer will have the time to explain why it may not be necessary. This is true for many treatments.

Physician's Perspective

When a mother comes to see me, wanting an antibiotic for her child's mild ear infection, I often don't have the time to explain all of the pros and cons. Part of my work, which I am attempting to change, is in a usual busy clinic that packs as many patients per unit time as possible. If there is time, I explain that, for a child more than two years of age, one needs to treat fifteen children in order to get relief of pain in one, and after treating twelve of them, at least one side-effect will be caused such as rash, diarrhea, or vomiting. There is usually insufficient time to speak about the development of resistant bacteria from frequent unnecessary antibiotics, effects of wiping out the beneficial intestinal flora, and the utility of affording a chance for the child's own immune system to take care of the problem. One is also faced with the possibility of being perceived by the patient as incompetent and uncaring, and losing the patient. Finally, one may want to maximize the placebo effect. It is well known that when the patient or those who are taking care of him believe that the treatment is beneficial, it works better. It is for this reason that good studies are double-blind (neither the patient nor his doctor knows whether the patient is getting a drug or a placebo). So when the mother really believes that amoxicillin (or some other drug) is sure to help her child, I usually give in (as do most other doctors), because it is more likely to help in that case.

Patient/Family Perspective

If you feel that you may be getting unnecessary tests and procedures, and for those who don't want to waste money, do not hesitate to ask the doctor why you need the test. If it is to rule out something that you are not likely to have—you are probably dealing with a doctor who wants to do the test just to comply with some standard. Don't become someone else's test animal, and a source of profit and reassurance. Sometimes the doctor may feel that by doing the test he will please you. This is not uncommon. There is some research that shows that patients feel better taken care of when more tests are done on them (Venning et al, 2000), and doctors are aware of that. In that situation, by questioning the test, you give that doctor a permission to say that additional tests are not really necessary. Ask the doctor how much benefit the risky treatment is likely to provide, before agreeing to it. Do your own research when possible; don't discount your own abilities to obtain information.

Surgery may involve complications in one or two percent of cases. That could possibly be you. Be sure that this risk is acceptable and worthwhile for you. If not, seek non-surgical alternatives.

Having read this far, do you still want more tests and procedures? I recommend the following to you. First, reconsider whether you really need more tests. If a physician in the US did not offer it himself, you probably do not need it. Here, we do too many tests as it is. If you insist, you'll probably get the test you want. You may be bothered by some unexplained symptom. Instead of asking for some test, ask to be referred to a specialist, if necessary seeking a second opinion after that. However, be prepared to stop and not to get into an endless cycle of doctor shopping. In spite of the common belief to the contrary, it is very common to never find an explanation for a symptom. I see several patients every week whose symptom of chest pain, headache, abdominal pain, or fatigue could not be explained by any physical finding by me, by the specialist, or by the tests. This is the rule rather than exception, and one that you don't see emphasized on TV. In addition, conditions such as irritable bowel syndrome, migraine, chronic back pain, chronic pelvic pain, chronic fatigue syndrome, fibromyalgia, are all names for the pains that medicine cannot fully explain. This does not mean that there is no treatment for this symptom, it just means that there is no medical test that will tell you what it is, only those that will tell you what it is not; usually there is no need to go through all of them.

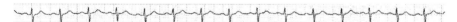

18

The Case of Unreason-able Expectations, Family Guilt and Blame

Patient/Family Perspective

This next incident happened when I was in my second year of residency. A seventy-eight year old woman was brought to the hospital by her son because of worsening swelling on her legs to the point that she wasn't able to care for herself. She was a very pleasant old lady and told us that she had not been feeling well for the past several months. Her son was adamant about our finding out and explaining to him what was going on with his mother, which we said we would do. He also wanted to know the prognosis. We told him that first we'd need to find out what was going on.

Several days went by and a large number of tests. No results were yielded by an echocardiogram (ultrasound of the heart), doppler studies of the leg veins, CT scan of the abdomen and pelvis, ultrasound of the liver. The patient's edema was worsening to the point that we now called it anasarca. She was swollen head to toe, with some fluid in the abdomen and chest. Blood tests showed somewhat low albumin, mild anemia, mild insufficiency of the kidneys, but failed to reveal the diagnosis. Some of the invasive tests were not done because of the risk of complications and low likelihood of cure. The patient's mental status was waxing and waning, and we continued doing more tests. We asked for a cardiology consultation. In the meantime we treated her with ever increasing doses of diuretics to get rid of some of the accumulated fluid. Gastroenterology and cardiology consultations did not help and the patient was becoming more anemic. There were multiple possibilities including gastrointestinal bleeding.

A week went by, and the patient's son did not get the answers he was hoping for. At this point we approached him and offered him the option of taking his mother back home, as it seemed less and less likely that we would be able to help this elderly and debilitated woman. If he didn't feel comfortable taking her home, we proposed an option of either aggressive further treatment and more tests, or supportive care only and a hospice placement. This made him feel very uncomfortable. He was openly angry about the lack of answers and accused us of incompetence. He got into frequent disputes with the nurses who were taking care of his mother. He told us that, if he knew that she only had a few more weeks to live, he would have taken her home. On the other hand, if this could last for a year, he'd have to accept a nursing home placement. He understandably hesitated and was very angry about the lack of definitive answers. When he asked a doctor who was covering for me over the weekend, the doctor told him that his mother was not likely to have more than a few weeks. The patient's son then asked for decreased intervention and no more blood tests. He hesitated between taking her home or arranging for a hospice care.

The following week, the patient felt worse and became more short of breath. Her son authorized a blood test that, together with a chest X-ray, showed that her anemia had worsened and the fluid in her lungs had increased. We raised the question of either a blood transfusion or palliative care. The son was in agony, trying to decide what to do. Neither the specialists nor our supervising physician could give him the answers he was seeking. On the one hand, he had the option of taking his mother home and taking care of her there with the help of home care nurses. On the other hand, he was afraid of making this step if something else could be done at the hospital; he also felt that he wouldn't want to take his mother home long-term, and he would feel bad sending her to the nursing home from his home later.

If a blood transfusion was to be done, the patient needed a central line, a kind of intravenous line used to access large veins in the neck, chest or groin. This is somewhat invasive and unpleasant. The patient herself delegated decision-making capacity to her son, feeling that he would know what was best. On Friday of the second week of her stay, the patient's son asked me if there was a possibility of her surviving long-term, to which I responded that there was. He than spoke with his mother and told us to proceed with the central line placement and blood transfusion, which we did. When I returned to the hospital on the following Monday, I found out that the patient passed away over the weekend. It seemed that she had an upper gastrointestinal bleeding and passed away quickly after vomiting some blood.

The son was furious and felt that he had been misled. Had he known that his mother was to die so soon, he would have taken her home and let her die there as she'd wanted. When I called him later that day to express my condolences and asked if he had questions, he responded with that he would keep questions for later—for the court (which thankfully didn't take place).

I decided to bring up this story for several reasons. One is to show that, unlike what is seen on TV (as in the ER series for example), there are still many cases when the answers cannot be found, even when we use the best of the modern technology. When answers are lacking, one needs to make decisions in the face of uncertainty. In this case, the patient's son hesitated for a week about taking his mother home. He was prepared to take care of her short term but could not accept the possibility that she could turn into a long term burden. I think he felt guilty about this, and this may explain his hostility towards the doctors and nurses. Uncertainty took him by surprise and got the best of him.

The medical system acted appropriately in this case, but the patient's son felt that it left him to deal with too difficult an issue. It is the disappointed belief that medicine will have all the necessary answers that frustrated this patient's son. *The lack of the doctor's ability to provide the diagnosis and to predict the timeframe of his mother's death disturbed him deeply.* He was unprepared for the following two facts. First, the medical system cannot give all the answers. Second, the medical system cannot make decisions for the patient or for his family. Expecting from the medical system to do these things is a mistake.

I hope I would not be disappointed, if I faced a similar situation with my own family. Generally speaking, if initial testing fails to yield clear answers for an elderly and sick patient, then doing more is very unlikely to help in improving the condition, even if the diagnosis is established in the end. Trying to guess how much longer the person has to live is not likely to be accurate. Developing your own sense of the patient's prognosis may help you in deciding how aggressive to be in managing a very ill loved-one. Ask yourself two questions: Is the person *old*, and is he or she *very sick?* If the answer to both is "yes", I would recommend avoiding any investigation or treatment that can bring harm, or even discomfort.

Not many doctors know how to help the family with these decisions. Many, as I have observed, will be afraid to give an assurance that it is acceptable to refuse further investigation or treatment. The opposite is more likely. Health professionals feel more comfortable doing more tests and more treatments. Sometimes this is because of their own unpreparedness to handle death; other times it may be the way they try to express that they care, but more often it is because of the fear of being sued later by the family. They fear that the family may later decide that more should have been done. If the family will not take the nonaggressive non-interventional initiative, it is likely that no one will.

The next step is usually deciding on the place for the patient—a nursing home, an inpatient or outpatient hospice, or at home with the family. I think that any decision is better than letting a significant amount of time lapse in indecision. When possible, consulting with other family members can be helpful. During such a discussion it is important not to assign blame or act out of guilt. This is harmful for both the patient and the family. Instead, accept your limitations and do what is possible in the moment.

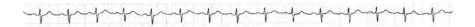

19 The Case of Letting Go

Patient/Family Perspective

This was a patient whom I admitted recently while being on call for one of my call group associates. It was an eighty-two year old woman brought to the ER by her husband. She'd had a major stroke two months prior, and her husband cared for her at home. After the stroke she became bed bound, with minimal ability to speak and some difficulties swallowing. She was also a diabetic. The husband brought her because she had an episode of choking, followed by shortness of breath while he was spoon feeding her. When I came to examine this patient, she was unable to speak; her eyes were open, but she didn't seem to realize what was happening to her. Her breathing improved after several bouts of coughing in the emergency room. Initial chest X-ray and blood tests looked OK. It was clear that she must have aspirated some of the food she ate, a very common complication after a stroke.

Further examination revealed a bed sore on her back that went down to the bone. This also happens often with elderly patients after a stroke, especially when they become bed bound and have trouble eating. The patient did not respond to my questions, did not try to communicate to me otherwise, or to resist my exam. The patient's husband was there and I couldn't help a deep sense of admiration for this elderly man. Two months prior, after she had a major stroke, he took her back home and spoon fed her, tried to do physical therapy for her, and changed dressings on her bed sore. A visiting nurse came three times a week; he took care of his wife the rest of the time. I spoke with him after examining his wife. He was obviously distraught by this turn of events. He told me that over the previous week his wife's verbal and mental responsiveness as well as her ability to move have been declining.

Physician's Perspective

A speech therapist came by to evaluate the patient's ability to swallow. She reported to me that the patient was not able to swallow at all and that officially she had to state that the patient was not a candidate for oral feeding. She also told me "we're supposed to tell about tube feeding, the nasogastric tube and the PEG tube" (one that goes through the abdominal wall directly into the stomach). She told me that she didn't think that the tube would be the right thing to do for this patient but she felt she could not tell this directly to the patient's husband. This is a very common phenomenon. All ancillary staff at the hospital are specifically taught defensive medicine by the hospital. They call it 'risk management.' If a speech therapist makes a mistake, it is the hospital, not the speech therapist that will be sued, because the speech therapist is a hospital employee. Hospitals therefore insure themselves by guiding their workers to carry out defensive practices. I told the speech therapist that, from my research, I did not find any evidence for using any kind of feeding tubes in old patients with severely diminished mental capacity. As I mentioned earlier in this book, ("The Case of Threatening the Doctor") these tubes will not prevent aspiration, will not increase comfort, will not prolong life, and are associated with their own adverse effects; especially so in the very frail patient.

I asked the speech therapist what kind of diet would be the least harmful, if offered in spite of patient's apparent inability to swallow. As with most tests, the swallowing test is not 100% accurate. Some of the patients who don't pass it are still able to swallow safely. She responded that she could not write this down in the chart, since it would appear that she authorized feeding the patient, but verbally she gladly told me to offer puree with nectar thick liquids.

The speech therapist acted here just as many doctors do. She was not willing to make a recommendation that was the right thing to do but was risky. The risk was serious—the patient could aspirate again, get aspiration pneumonia and die. The benefit of allowing the patient to eat was avoiding the suffering associated with tube placement and maintenance, and the possibility of the patient tolerating the meal in spite of the failed swallowing test and enjoying the meal. Death was a risk whether the tube was placed or not. Putting in the tubes was not going to help this patient, but at least the health care providers would be able to say that everything possible was done and thus would feel protected in court. One humane option would be to allow her gently starve to death. There is no discomfort after the first few days ('starvation euphoria' will be discussed later), and this lady was already malnourished, so perhaps there'd be no hunger pangs at all. Another humane option would be to let her eat, if she expressed the wish to do so, and accept the possibility of her dying of an aspiration pneumonia.

Patient/Family Perspective

When I spoke to the patient's husband, he was already convinced by the speech therapist of the need for the tube. I described to him the downside of having the tube placed, and he agreed to wait until the next day, when he could discuss this again with his wife's regular doctor for whom I was covering. The husband also was very concerned about the patient's inability to take her diabetic pills. Her blood sugars ranged around 200mg/dL, and he felt this was doing her harm. I explored this idea with him further. We spoke about the importance of keeping blood sugar under control long term, but I told him that for the moment, in his wife's situation, it was not of major importance. While to me it seemed clear that his wife was dying, he seemed unprepared to face this. He asked me about the prognosis and I told him that I did not think it was good. I recommended that he would also speak about this with his wife's doctor. From our short conversation, I gathered that he had developed a good relationship with their doctor. It seemed that their doctor would have been a better person to address issues of end of life care.

Physician's Perspective

I continued stopping by to check the patient's progress after her doctor took over. I was happy to see that a tube was not placed, and her doctor did start her on a pureed diet, which the patient was tolerating for the moment. A consultation from a wound care specialist stated that the prognosis for wound healing was *exceptionally poor,* but he surgically débrided it anyway (cut out pieces of dead tissue) and proposed a course of treatment. I later inquired about this patient from her doctor. The doctor told me that after spending a few weeks at a nursing home the patient was back in the hospital. The husband was not ready to let her go, and the doctor, at his request, consulted a gastroenterologist for placing a PEG tube (a tube that goes through the abdominal wall directly into the stomach) to feed the patient that way.

Patient/Family Perspective

To have sent her to the nursing home was a reasonable, but not the only option. She could have been allowed to die at home. A dying patient does not need aggressive wound care, strict management of diabetes, or physical therapy. One way of seeing this situation is that a nursing home could care for her better before she succumbed to infection, malnutrition, or pneumonia; another way to see this is that she would suffer more by spending her last days in an unfamiliar environment, confused, and "treated" (and re-hospitalized and sometimes even placed into an intensive care unit) for what is an inevitable and natural course of events. Even in a nursing home, there is usually an option of signing a 'Do Not Hospitalize' directive, along with 'Do Not Resuscitate' and 'Do Not Intubate.' 'No Antibiotics', 'No Intravenous Fluids', and 'No Tube Feeding' are other directives that can help one have a more humane end. To be able to explore that, the family member has to be able to handle the passing of a loved one and be prepared to let go. He or she has to overcome the belief that less medical care equals to less caring. He or she actually needs to be the one to initiate this conversation. The medical team may fail to do so, and by default the patient will suffer from every possible unnecessary medical intervention.

Societal Perspective

Less than one fourth of seriously ill patients talk to their physicians about their preferences for end of life care. A study done in 1997 shows that for most patients, as for most physicians, this is an uncomfortable topic. Many of the patients who did not discuss their preferences did not want aggressive measures (Hofmann et al, 1997). The authors of the study concluded, "For patients who do not want to discuss their preferences, as well as patients with an unmet need for such discussions, failure to discuss preferences for cardiopulmonary resuscitation and mechanical ventilation may result in unwanted interventions." In fact, unwanted interventions are an everyday reality. People who do not discuss their preferences about end of life care with their health care providers are probably not very clear about that with their family members. Most of them end up getting all kinds of medical interventions before they die.

Most people in the US prefer to die at home, but in fact most die at a hospital (Pritchard et al, 1998). A review of data from seventy-seven hospitals in the 2001 *US News and World Report* 'best hospitals' list for heart and pulmonary disease, cancer, and geriatric services shows the following (Wennberg et al, 2004): In the last six months of life, 9-27 days (ranges between different hospital averages) were spent in the hospital, 2-9 days were spent in the intensive care unit of a hospital, there were 17-76 doctor visits, 16-58% of patients were seen by more than 10 doctors, 15-55% died in the hospital and 8-36% in the intensive care unit. I do not think that many of us would want to spend our last six months attended by ten or more different doctors, spending any time in the intensive care unit, and dying at the hospital. To be sure, the more doctors you have, the more tests and treatments you are likely to get, even more so when you are hospitalized, and still more when in the intensive care unit. The costs, of course, are huge.

A study points out that "the risk of in-hospital death was increased for residents of regions with greater hospital bed availability and use; the risk of in-hospital death was decreased in regions with greater nursing home and hospice availability and use. Measures of hospital bed availability and use were the most powerful predictors of place of death across Hospital Referral Regions" (Pritchard et al, 1998). To me this means that patients and their families have delegated the decision-making process to the doctors, who then assumed that the family is not able to care for the patient and send the patient wherever there is room. Hospice care is mainly a form of home care, although there are inpatient hospices as well. They can provide a wide range of palliative care, some of which I will discuss in the next chapter.

There is now data confirming what before was only an educated guess—that higher intensity of care in the last six months of life does not prolong, but actually shortens life. A review of US healthcare put together by Dartmouth Medical School states: "Indeed, greater intensity of care, measured by use of intensive care units, was actually associated with a slight increase in mortality, a finding compatible with the hypothesis that more intervention is actually associated with worse outcomes. Moreover, most patients appear to prefer less intensive care at the end of life, and those who live in regions with lower intensity of care are more likely to receive the care they say they want (which is generally less than most people now receive). It is reasonable to use those regions in which the intensity of end of life care is low as "best practice" benchmarks of efficiency, because in those areas, lower spending results in no known loss of benefit, and appears to reflect actual patient preferences for end of life care. Three hospital referral regions provide such benchmarks for the use of intensive care in the last six months of life: Sun City, Arizona, Portland, Oregon, and Minneapolis" (The Dartmouth Atlas of Health Care 1999, excerpted with permission).

So most of us want less intervention in the last six months of our lives, but we end up getting more and without any benefit. Why? Some ideas come from an analysis of this issue in the Dartmouth Atlas project, which is a funded research effort of the faculty of the Center for the

Evaluative Clinical Sciences at Dartmouth Medical School to study the health care system in the United States. "The quality of medical intervention is often more a matter of the quality of caring than the quality of curing, and never more so than when life nears its end. Yet medicine's focus is disproportionately on curing, or at least on the ability to keep patients alive with life-support systems and other medical interventions. This ability to intervene at the end of life has raised a host of medical and ethical issues for patients, physicians, and policy makers." I think that this problem can be addressed by patients and their families, if they realize in advance the difference between caring and curing. While in order to cure one needs to care, the reverse is not true. Cure cannot be forced; otherwise it results in more suffering.

"More than 80% of patients say that they wish to avoid hospitalization and intensive care during the terminal phase of illness, but those wishes are often overridden by other factors...More intense intervention does not improve life expectancy...Most patients prefer less care when more intensive care is likely to be futile..." The question then becomes how to determine where that cutoff point is, when the aggressive care becomes futile. The answer, in my opinion, is that there is absolutely no way of knowing that with certainty. Yet, leaving this important part of our lives unattended clearly brings more suffering. As in all other uncertain medical matters, one must decide what the cutoff point would be. It could be a certain age, certain degree of mental or physical decline, certain degree of loss of capacity to care for self or many other criteria. But if people does not make this choice for themselves they are in effect choosing the default way, which is usually the way of unnecessary suffering before dying.

A large study (Anonymous, 1995) undertook to improve end-of-life decision making by studying it and then intervening. "A specifically trained nurse had multiple contacts with the patient, family, physician, and hospital staff to elicit preferences, improve understanding of outcomes, encourage attention to pain control, and facilitate advance care planning and patient-physician communication." This intervention failed to improve outcomes; the same percentages of patients who wished to die at home ended up receiving many interventions and dying in the hospital. Why? The authors of the study give their hypothesis:

"Probably the best explanation is that the local supply of hospital resources, and local physicians' practice styles, are far more dominant determinants of how care is given at the end of life than either patient preferences or the best clinical strategies to avoid unwelcome interventions. The SUPPORT study took place at five different hospitals in five different hospital referral regions. The percent of study patients who died in hospitals ranged from a low of 29% to a high of 66%. The variations were not explained by sociodemographic characteristics, clinical profiles, or patients' preferences" (excerpted with permission from The Dartmouth Atlas of Health Care, 1999).

A recent study (Wennberg et al, 2004) came to the same conclusion as an earlier one (Pritchard, 1998) which discovered, that the industry determines how we die, or the local availability of beds. "Among regions, a direct relation exists between supply and utilization of services. The frequency of use of physician services is strongly associated with the local workforce supply, and bed supply "explains" more than half of the variation in hospital admission rates for medical conditions. The effect of bed supply is to influence the threshold for admitting patients with chronic illnesses such as congestive heart failure, chronic pulmonary obstructive disease, and cancer. Finally, physicians have been shown to adapt their decisions about admission and discharge to the availability of intensive care unit beds, admitting more patients with lower severity of illness and extending their length of stay when more beds are available. In the light of this evidence, the likely explanation for the variations in acute hospital care and physician visits is variation in bed and workforce capacity relative to the size of population loyal to the seventy-seven hospitals."

This availability varies among different regions and seems to mirror the concentration of the elderly. In other words, the business finds its way to where there is demand. More hospital beds and more ICU beds are created where there are more potential customers—dying people—Florida, California, Texas. See the figures created by The Dartmouth Atlas of Health Care (1999) on the following pages.

"The place of death and the intensity of interventions provided depend much more on the region's patterns of use of acute care hospital resources than on what dying patients say that they want." The findings indicated that neither patient preferences nor Medicare spending were predictive of the intensity of care patients were going to get. In fact, spending predicted increased intensity of treatments as did the availability of beds. What seems to happen is that as soon as there is a large concentration of the elderly, the business of medicine moves in under the pretext of trying to provide *adequate care to the community*. Hospital beds and jobs are created, then a practice pattern is established in order to justify their existence. This practice pattern leads to a lot more interventions without any benefit. "…the evidence…characterizes a system in which large amounts

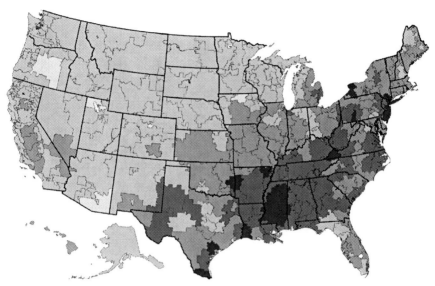

**Percent of Medicare Deaths
Occurring in Hospitals**

by Hospital Referral Region (1995-96)

■	40 or More	(24)
■	35 to < 40	(67)
■	30 to < 35	(102)
▨	20 to < 30	(108)
□	Less than 20	(5)
▨	Not Populated	

**Fig. 19-1 Percent of Medicare Deaths Occurring in Hospitals
(1995-96)**

Reproduced with permission. Copyright the Trustees of Dartmouth College, 1999.

"Medicare enrollees who lived in the Eastern and Southern United States were more likely to die as hospital inpatients than residents of the Western and Northwestern parts of the country. Rates were particularly high in the New York-New Jersey metropolitan area and in Mississippi, and much lower than average in Tucson, Arizona; Ogden, Utah; Bend, Oregon; and Mason City, Iowa."

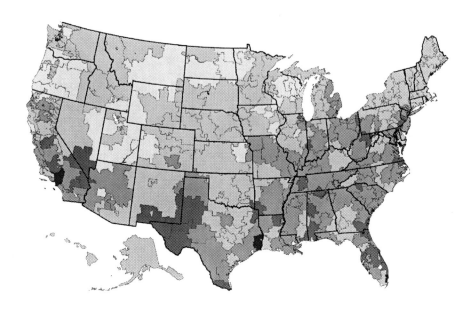

**Percent of Medicare Enrollees Who
Spent Seven or More Days in Intensive
Care During the Last Six Months of Life**

by Hospital Referral Region (1995-96)

- 20 or More   (4)
- 15 to < 20   (35)
- 10 to < 15   (115)
-   5 to < 10   (128)
- Less than 5   (24)
- Not Populated

**Fig. 19-2 Percent of Medicare Enrollees Who Spent 7 or More Days
in Intensive Care During Their Last 6 Months of Life (1995-96)**

Reproduced with permission. Copyright the Trustees of Dartmouth College, 1999.

"The likelihood of spending at least one week of the last six months of
life in intensive care was higher among enrollees in the East, Midwest,
Texas and southern California. Medicare residents of the Upper Midwest,
Mountain states, and Oregon were on average less likely to spend seven or
more days in intensive care at the end of life."

of money are spent on medical intervention that provides no benefit, whether that benefit is measured in longevity or in honoring patients' preferences."

Below are the worst and the best regions, respectively, for end-of-life. The worst places to die are the following "…18 hospital referral regions, [where] the likelihood of one or more admissions to intensive care during the last six months of life was greater than 40%, including Miami (49.3%); Munster, Indiana (48.7%); Los Angeles (45.8%); St. Petersburg, Florida (44.2%); Beaumont, Texas (43.9%); and Newark, New Jersey (43.9%)."

The following are the best places to be for a more peaceful death: "In ten hospital referral regions, the likelihood of admission to intensive care during the last six months of life was less than 20%, including Sun City, Arizona (14.2%); Bloomington, Illinois (15.2%); Bend, Oregon (16.6%); Wausau, Wisconsin (16.9%); Mason City, Iowa (16.9%); and Grand Junction, Colorado (17.4%)" (Excerpted with permission from: The Dartmouth Atlas of Health Care 1999).

But this is not the whole story. This only describes the environment. While we cannot control our environment we can control our choices. The following excerpt indicates that in the end we make the choice that results in this unnecessary suffering. "The vast majority—82% reported that if a doctor told them they had "very little time to live," they would prefer death at home, rather than in a hospital. In most cases, however, those who die do not know with certainty that they will die within a certain time frame. Different people might place different degrees of importance on the (perhaps small) chance of surviving, versus the discomforts and risks of high-technology interventions. Some people die in intensive care units not because they prefer them to other settings, but because they were willing to take the risk of intense intervention in exchange for the chance of recovery."

Patient/Family Perspective

There are two important points that can be addressed here. One is the delegation of responsibility to the doctor. Patients believe that doctor will know more about them than they know about themselves. They hope that the doctor will tell them when they have "very little time to live." Such an expectation is unreasonable for a number of reasons. The doctor cannot really know for sure when someone will die. A premature statement could lead to a self-fulfilling prophecy. A person might recover if given hope, die if told that is the most likely. Even when the prognosis seems clear to the doctor, he is often afraid to tell this to the patient. The doctor may feel that the patient does not want to hear it, he or she may be afraid of possible legal repercussions; or because a physician is inextricably tied into the system within which he or she is working often to the point of carrying out decisions automatically and without much awareness following the so called community standard.

The second point is that, when we are ill, we are faced with a temptation to believe that the high-technology may save us. We then put our faith into it while trying to cling to life at all costs. It is the last step where we could prevent some suffering, if we could stop ourselves from this excessive clinging. We could reduce some of our suffering by letting go of the excessive fear of death, and of the belief that high technology can save us.

I hope that if my loved ones would have to face a similar situation, they would not put their faith in doctors and would not be tempted by high technology. Instead, accepting the situation as it is and realizing that no one else knows what is best for them, I hope they would not cling to physical existence at any cost. I hope that when the time comes, they will be able to go preserving their human dignity and inner peace.

Below is a table listing the top ten causes of death in the US in 1900, 1950, and 2000 (CDC/NCHS). Note that pneumonia, for instance, while jumping from the first to the sixth place from 1900 to 1950, since then descended only one more step, being now the seventh leading cause of death.

1900	1950	2000
1) Pneumonia (all forms) and influenza	1) Diseases of heart	1) Diseases of heart
2) Tuberculosis (all forms)	2) Cancer	2) Cancer
3) Diarrhea, enteritis, and ulceration of the intestines	3) Cerebrovascular disease	3) Cerebrovascular diseases
4) Diseases of the heart	4) Accidents (MVA and other)	4) Chronic lower respiratory diseases
5) Cerebrovascular disease	5) Certain diseases of early infancy	5) Accidents (unintentional injuries)
6) Kidney disease	6) Influenza and pneumonia	6) Diabetes mellitus
7) All accidents	7) Tuberculosis, all forms	7) Influenza and pneumonia
8) Cancer	8) General arteriosclerosis	8) Alzheimer's disease
9) Senility	9) Kidney disease	9) Kidney disease
10) Diphtheria	10) Diabetes mellitus	10) Septicemia

Table 19-1: Top Ten Causes Of Death In The US (source: CDC/NCHS)

Spiritual/Philosophical Perspective

Dr. Gerald N. Epstein, who is a psychiatrist and a practitioner of what he calls western spiritual medicine, writes the following with respect to putting one's faith in the wrong thing:

"The antibiotic: the patient is given the pills and after two weeks the pneumonia clears up. Again, another idolatrous statement is made by the doctor: "The antibiotic cured you." If you buy that conclusionary comment, you begin putting your faith in a pill to the point of worshipping this little white pill" (Epstein, 2004).

While it is true that the pill (the antibiotic in this case) is helpful, to believe that it is responsible for a cure is an enormous mistake. If it were so, pneumonia wouldn't still be the seventh leading cause of death in the US, or as they say—"an old man's friend." The antibiotic, at best, helps the body do its own work of curing, and when the body gives up, as is seen in the very elderly and in immuno-compromised patients, no amount of antibiotic will save a person. In the realms dealing with life and death, the medical-scientific axis crosses the philosophical-spiritual axis. On this note we will continue to the last chapter, which deals with preparedness for death.

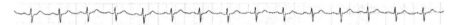

20 Freedom in Living and in Dying

Spiritual/Philosophical Perspective

While healthy optimism is essential for recovery, excessive attachment to the physical, as described in the previous chapter, increases misery without prolonging life. Seduced by the temptation that comes from the current medical system, we fall victim to someone else's increased profits. As long as we have this exaggerated belief in the capabilities of high technology, we will be vulnerable to anyone who pretends to hand out immortality under the name of another new drug or a new procedure. We are terrified of death and are afraid of even speaking about it. Paralyzed by this fear, we end up in the hands of death unprepared, clinging and quivering, often in agony and sometimes in despair. I think that being ready to face death is essential for both the patient who is seriously ill, and for the family members taking care of that patient. Once this fear is faced, we are no longer so easily seduced by the false promises and gain some degree of freedom while alive and when dying.

During my short medical career, I've witnessed a number of deaths (mainly during my residency), and participated in the resuscitation efforts of a number of patients. I got to know two of those patients quite well. In addition, prior to medical school I worked as a nurse, caring for the dying in a nursing home and doing home care. It has never been easy, but it is not as gloomy a process as it is usually painted. I think that one way to approach the experience of death is to speak of palliative care.

I would encourage anyone to read the rest of this chapter without skipping or running through quickly. Those who are seriously ill may find some consolation that medicine can provide certain comfort when used appropriately, even at the time of death. Death itself is not a pathologic process or something to be ashamed of. Viewing death as a failure is a by-product of the industrial age with its arrogant implied presupposition that technological advances can make us immortal. This is acknowledged in an article on palliative care. "The dramatic advances in medical care that have taken place during the past century have had the untoward side effect of changing the definition of death from the natural culmination of life into an unwanted outcome of disease and a failure of medical intervention" (Meier, 1998).

Palliative care is medical care directed at providing comfort measures and not on curing the disease. It is an intervention intended to immediately improve comfort without long term goals. As defined by the World Health Organization, palliative care is the active total care of a patient whose disease does not respond to curative treatment. Control of pain, of other symptoms, and of psychological, social, and spiritual problems is paramount. The goal of palliative care is the achievement of the best quality of life that is possible for the patient and the family. Hospice care can assist the family in caring for the dying. It consists of a team of a physician, nurses, home health aids, a social worker, a physical therapist, and others. The usual hospice benefit covers four hours of home aid and the family is expected to take care of the patient the other twenty hours a day.

Among the common symptoms that can be helped with palliative measures are pain, fatigue, dry mouth, constipation, nausea, vomiting, diarrhea, shortness of breath, cough, anxiety and confusion. One article on palliative care also lists poor appetite as a symptom that can be helped (Montagnini, 2004). This deserves a moment of attention. Obviously when a dying person communicates, it is easier to ascertain whether he or she is bothered by hunger or other sensations. For those who are no longer able to communicate, we often try to guess how to make them more comfortable. It is common to assume for both the family and the health care workers that poor appetite or inability to eat needs to be remedied, possibly because it will bring a discomfort of feeling hungry. This idea sometimes leads to insistent feeding, and feeding tube placement. It is important to realize that this idea is an assumption. If a dying person does not want to eat, there is no reason to try to feed him or her either by giving appetite increasing medications or tube feedings. In fact, there is good evidence of something called "starvation euphoria" which is a very comfortable state experienced after some degree of starvation by chronically seriously ill patients (Truog et al., 2001). Body chemistry changes and one is naturally made comfortable. By force-feeding we may be removing the possibility of this comfort and adding new discomforts.

Pain may accompany the dying process and medication can be given to reduce it. Opiate medications are available in forms of pills, liquid, lollypops, rectal suppositories, injectables, and nebulized for inhalation. Multiple side-effects can be encountered from the use of these drugs, some of which can be bothersome and require treatment. Most notably, for some, these medications can cause mental confusion. Other side effects include constipation, nausea and vomiting, dry mouth, urinary retention, low blood pressure, risk of falls, and respiratory suppression. How aggressively these need to be managed depends on whether the dying person is bothered by them, and the length of time the treatment is given. Respiratory suppression from these drugs is accompanied by a diminished feeling of shortness of breath. This is used as a palliative measure by itself for those patients who are suffering from feeling of shortness of breath. The use of opiates for this purpose may be in addition to oxygen, anti-anxiety medications, and corticosteroids. Opioids are also used for cough suppression. The other side-effects of the narcotics such as nausea and vomiting, constipation, urinary retention can be managed with other medications. The medications used also have side effects.

Dementia with delirium, anxiety and mental confusion can be helped with some medications. They may be the result of some of the natural processes, as well as a side effect of certain medications used for pain control, or for many other purposes. Some medications that can have mental side-effects include those used for anxiety, fatigue, urinary retention, and some of the anti-nausea medications.

Dry mouth occurs frequently, and usually is a side effect of a medication. It can make speaking and swallowing more difficult. Sips of water, hard candy, and medications (again not without side-effects) can be used.

Feeling of fatigue can be a part of a natural physical or mental process or a side effect of a medication (opiates and other pain relieving drugs, some blood pressure drugs and others). Steroids and stimulants can be used, each with their own set of side-effects. In the article I used as a reference (Montagnini, MD, 2004) treatment of anemia and poor appetite is recommended. This may be a reasonable option for someone who wishes to stay active and is bothered by fatigue. It may be appropriate for a person who wants to complete a project requiring energy and sustained attention. Injectable medications can improve anemia in those cases without the need for a blood transfusion, and appetite stimulants can improve appetite. Of course, as the number of medications increases, one can reach a point where the problems they cause equal or exceed the suffering that patient would naturally experience. Balance needs to be found.

In the final stages, the person may be too weak to spit or swallow their saliva, which then collects deep in the throat and produces noisy breathing known as "death rattle." This is known to occur in about 25% of the dying. While medications and other medical measures are available, one needs to recognize the point where one is no longer treating the dying person's discomfort but one's own difficulty coping with the process of dying. Ask yourself whether it is the dying person who is suffering from this process (such as a death rattle) or is it I who is having trouble hearing it. If it bothers you but there is no clear indication that it bothers the dying person, there is no need to try to treat it. Instead, try to accept it and if you cannot, step outside and let someone else care for the dying until you regain your strength.

In our western society, we are generally uncomfortable approaching death. Some eastern thought can be helpful as described in the *Tibetan Book of Living and Dying* (Rinpoche, 1993). Tibetans give much thought, importance and preparation to the process of dying. They believe that even a person who lived life in error can achieve salvation during the process of dying. The author of the book, a Tibetan monk, recommends dying at home when possible, where familiar surroundings will provide for a more peaceful state of mind. When this is not possible and the person will be dying in the hospital or nursing home, he recommends bringing plants, flowers, pictures and photographs of the loved ones, drawings by children and grandchildren, audio of favorite music and when possible home-cooked meals. He also recommends that the family should address the need for tests and injections as these can provoke anger, irritation and pain, and for the Tibetan a peaceful state of mind at the time of death is of great importance. A Buddhist spiritual master of eighth century, Shanti-deva said:

> *"If all the harms*
> *Fears and sufferings in the world*
> *Arise from self-grasping,*
> *What need have I for such a great evil spirit?"*

Indeed it is this self-grasping that not only misleads us into excessive utilization of medical services, but also brings suffering in our last moments, when instead of staying with the moment and receiving it as is, we seek to change, to mold, hang on to, so that our self would remain the same, not changed by what comes. This clinging to the idea of how things should be improved leads to much additional suffering. Readily accepting what the moment brings, without the preconceived ideas of how things should or could be, makes for a much smoother transition.

The author of the book, Sogyal Rinpoche, says that the Buddhist attitude toward death can be summed up by one verse from the *Tibetan Book of the Dead*:

"Now when the [painful reality of dying] dawns upon me,
I will abandon all grasping, yearning and attachment,
Enter undistracted into clear awareness of the [spiritual] teaching,
And eject my consciousness into the space of [the One mind/Holy spirit];
As I leave this compound body of flesh and blood
I will know to be a transitory illusion."

The importance of abandoning grasping, yearning and attachment is emphasized again. When this attitude is adopted, the mind may be at peace and crystal clear. One then knows what to do in the moment and is unafraid.

Western spiritual tradition (Judaism, Christianity, and Islam) offers some tools that may be easier to understand for the westerner. Reading the twenty third psalm of the Bible, for instance, can remove fear. It needs not be attempted with a person who has unresolved religious conflicts. A mental exercise may be helpful for those who are inclined to try that kind of work. This work was developed by Colette Aboulker-Muscat and Dr. Gerald N. Epstein. It permits one to tap into one's inner resources rather than looking for an external figure (such as a physician) to provide relief from mental suffering through medication. To do it, a participant is asked to close his or her eyes and breathing out three times slowly (making normal inhalation and slow long exhalations). A participant is given the following instructions:

Imagine yourself carrying your rod and staff.

Use your staff to help you walk a straight road, and use your rod to knock away any fearful image that intrudes on your path.

Then see your cup overflowing.

Open your eyes, knowing that your fear has gone.

This mental exercise may help relieve the fear of pain, suffering, and dying, and bring calmness with greater clarity of consciousness.

Another mental exercise may be of help to anyone faced with a difficult decision but particularly a seriously ill person trying to decide on a course medical care. It also comes from a book by Dr. Gerald N. Epstein (Epstein, 1999).

"Close your eyes, breathe out three times, and imagine yourself standing behind a golden balance scale with two golden balance pans.

Have with you a pad of white paper. On a slip of paper write an advantage or a positive aspect of one choice and put it on one pan. Continue writing the advantages of this choice, one per slip, and put them in the pan.

Then write the advantage or positive aspect of the other choice and put it on the other pan. Again, continue writing the advantages of this choice, one per slip, and put them in the pan.

See which pan weighs more, and open your eyes. Then immediately carry out the decision that the pans have indicated."

Sometimes we may be forced by circumstances to make decisions for someone else, because that person's state of mind no longer permits them decision making. Generally, it is helpful to have had a discussion in advance. Options include a living will—a written advance directive, or designating a health care proxy (a person, usually a relative, who has discussed the issue of end of life care with the patient in advance). This person is designated by the patient to make decisions on his behalf, should the patient lose decision-making capacity himself. In reality, this is not always possible, and family members are often caught by surprise. When making such decisions, a conference with other family members can be helpful if it can be done without provoking disputes.

Again a mental exercise may be helpful for some.

Close your eyes, breathe out three times slowly and imagine calling the soul of the dying relative to give you advice in this difficult decision that you are asked to make (for an atheist imagine the relative in his best potential with all the wisdom, knowledge, and understanding that he could have achieved in life while remaining himself).

With reverence and very politely ask what they would want done for themselves.

Hear the answer and thank them.

Breathe out, open your eyes and act immediately according to the instructions you received.

This is a very reliable method for someone the decision maker knows well such as a close relative.

I find some poems by Colette Aboulker-Muscat (Aboulker-Muscat, 1995, the first two poems are reproduced with permission from ACMI Press, the third poem, among others, was given to me by its author with all rights) who was, among other things, a spiritual guide and a teacher of mind-body medicine, helpful in approaching and facing death without fear, regret, or shame, but instead with contentment and readiness.

Order in Life

What may I want
Out of Life!
The True meaning?
If I may again
Live my life
What may I choose
To do this time?
The Ideas
That have been mine
Do I want now
For them to die?
What may bring more
Joy and freshness
Than anything else
In the world?
I have put order in my life
And may now sleep quietly
With those I love all around
And the only One.
High,
In sky.

Life

At every change
And every turn of life
We, behind us
Are leaving the past.
With wisdom, humor
And serenity.
As a ripe fruit
Falls from the tree
Blessing the Earth
That has fed it,
And giving thankful graces
To the tree, for being.

Death

If I want to revenge
I triumph of It.
If I am in love
I forget It.
If my honor is spoiled
I am calling for It.
If I am in despair
Death is protecting me.
If I am anxious,
In advance I live It.
Faith and Joy
Are embracing It,
Opening the door
Where together,
We are passing through.

The poetry speaks for itself.

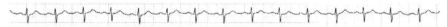

21 Putting It All Together: How To Get What You Want And Know What You Need

Patient/Family Perspective

Here I summarize all of the main points from the previous chapters for a quick review. After the book is read once, it is my hope that going over these last few pages will quickly refresh the entire content. This may be a useful ten minute reading prior to a discussion with a physician or before making a medical decision. All of the tools summarized here are intended to increase prospective patient's confidence, and help to achieve peace and clarity of mind.

Do not ignore your personal preferences. When you are given advice by a physician, be it in the examination room, emergency room, or a hospital, realize that this advice is rarely if ever tailored to you personally. Instead, it is usually a pre-programmed, automatic response based on an algorithm developed for treating patients with a similar set of problems. A physician cannot possibly know about you all that you know about yourself. Therefore, while the doctor may be doing his or her best, it may not always be what's best for you. Do not disregard your thoughts, feelings, and intuition when they do not go along with the doctor's advice. Instead, use them for further questioning, or if you feel you are hitting a wall, as a reason to seek another opinion, or stick to your own opinion.

Understand what goes into your doctor's decision-making process. While your doctor may attempt to do what is best for you, there are various pressures that he must deal with, and therefore has to juggle. After initial struggle, most doctors form a practice style whereby they act automatically and are no longer aware of this decision making process. Pressed by the legal fear, financial strain, practice guidelines, and bound by the medical model that cannot accept most patients as they are without assigning them to a category, they will usually act in a way that makes a compromise between all those pressures and the patient's interest. By taking this into account, one can understand better why a doctor may be insistent and may *want* you to do one thing or another. This gives a more realistic perspective on a physician, and his decision-making process.

Do the test only when you understand why you are doing it, and are prepared to deal with the consequences. Do not go along with what you are asked to do just to be nice to your doctor. There may be serious repercussions to your health. Before going for any test, ask what will be the next step, if the test comes back abnormal and if the test comes back normal. If it is not something you are prepared to go for (surgery, for example), there is no need for a test. Ask about the side effects of the test itself, before you decide (even seemingly benign tests, such as cardiac exercise stress testing, have side-effects). Do the test only if you understand why you are doing it, not just to follow what the doctor says.

Do not threaten the physician who is still taking care of you. This will usually lead to an increase in the defensive medicine which a lay person is not likely to recognize as such. Under the cover of "making sure" and "doing everything," many unnecessary tests and procedures will be done, and you or your loved one will suffer more. All this will be done to protect the doctor from a possible future lawsuit. If you feel dissatisfied with the care you're getting—have an open discussion with your doctor without any threats. If you must threaten, save it for the time when this doctor is no longer caring for you or your relative. Switch to a different doctor first.

Be sure that you understand recommendations of the specialists before accepting them. As with the tests, one needs to understand the reasons for consultations with specialists. Whether your doctor is referring you from the office or asking for a consultation while you are hospitalized, ask him what he hopes to achieve with a consultation, if it is not clear to you. At the end of the consultation do the following three things. 1) Clarify what tests, procedures, or treatments are recommended. 2) Clarify how the results of these tests or procedures are going to change the management of your condition and what will be the next step; for the treatments inquire how much difference the treatment is likely to make. 3) Clarify what the tests, procedures, or treatments entail, the side-effects, the degree of discomfort involved, the risks. Then make a decision whether to accept a recommendation or not. Do not offer yourself as a passive lamb to be sacrificed on the altar of "omnipotent," defensive medicine.

When in a situation involving end-of-life issues, be aware what going to the hospital and staying home (or in a nursing home) entails. If you go to the hospital, tests and procedures will be done, and they involve some discomfort and pain. An Emergency Room doctor will never say—"You need to go back home to die in peace." He or she will always assume that investigation and treatment are wanted, at least initially. If you stay at home, you have to be prepared to handle death. Comfort measures are better provided at home, by the family alone or with help of a hospice program or a physician. A nursing home is not as good as home, but usually is better than a hospital.

In issues of childbirth, as in other medical issues, an informed consent is not as informative as it may seem. If you are not satisfied with the options given, ask more questions. Ask what the actual risks are. The *absolute* risks are useful to know, not the relative increase or decrease of risk. For instance, don't accept a statement that the risk increases by 50%, doubles, or triples, but ask about the actual numbers. For instance, the data on the likelihood of a newborn baby having injury or death during the process of birthing increases in babies born vaginally in breech position. The risk is one in a hundred, versus one in a thousand if the baby is delivered by a cesarean section (Gifford et al, 1995). Most of this difference is due to injury (0.89%) not death (0.21%), with a total increase in the combined outcome of injury or death of 1.1%. Two things can be pointed out here. One is the usual practice of combining outcomes (such as injury and death in this case, where death is much less likely than injury); this combined number appears more impressive. The other point is the relative, versus absolute risk. The relative increase in risk is ten fold; and you will be told that you are increasing the likelihood of injuring the baby ten times if you go for a vaginal breech delivery. What you really need to know is the absolute numbers, which in this case is still very small, one percent. Also, remember that the study that found the increase can be altogether wrong.

Also, realize the limitations of medical science: what is considered good today may be discovered to be bad tomorrow. Understand that a doctor who is concerned about the risk of what you want to do, may be more concerned about the risk that it presents to him or her(in case of a future lawsuit) than the risk that it presents to you. For a pregnant woman who wants to have a vaginal delivery with a baby in breech position, if there is time, you need to inquire about doctors and midwifes who would do it. These are few, but they exist in some places. It is better to take care of this early in pregnancy. Ask a doctor what he would do if baby is in breech. If you want to try for a vaginal birth after a prior cesarean delivery, you may need to go to a larger university hospital, or otherwise find a practitioner who'd be willing to try.

If you feel you're being convinced, sold, or pressured—the doctor's motives are probably questionable. When being pressured, do not give in. Realize that doctors are pressured by the fear of lawsuits and by the medical industry through the guidelines, education, and legal system, to follow a certain pre-determined course of action. In the hospitals, institutional protocols are taking over parts of medical care. With the various pressures presented earlier in the book, your doctor may be less yours and more the industry's or hospital's or his own assets-protecting doctor. Smaller hospitals allow more flexibility but fewer specialists may be available when needed. The doctor's job is to explain evidence and risks, present the patient with options, answer questions, and give an opinion, not to convince the patient.

Be confident in your ability to decide correctly for yourself. If you feel that you know what to do, don't bother asking for opinions. If you need an opinion, it is better to ask a doctor when he is alone with you, so he would feel less pressured by his colleagues' presence to say "the right thing." If he says "it is recommended that…", or "according to the guidelines…" he is not telling you his opinion because of fear or for other reasons. Some may never reveal to you what they really think. Remember that you do not have to follow someone else's opinion. Be your own authority.

Beware of the hidden 'side-effects' of some treatments such as the time lost from your life to the multiple doctor and treatment visits. Time is precious. Have an active coping style, do not accept passively all that you are told, and do not follow blindly. When given a recommendation that is going to impact your quality of life, determine whether it is worth for you to follow it. Only you can determine how valuable certain aspects of your life are. Beware of treatments that significantly impact your life but may not be presented as side-effects. These are the time commitments that some treatments may require. This time will be taken from other important things in your life. Do not be surprised in the end if the time, supposedly the time that you've gained, has disappeared.

The medical system cannot fully explain, nor successfully treat all of your symptoms. If your symptom is bothersome and has not been explained, it may be reasonable to have an additional test, a consultation with a specialist, or to change a doctor, but do not fall into a cycle of endless search for explanations and reassurance. If you cannot stop yourself, the doctors are not likely to stop you. This involves too much of a risk for the doctor. If you keep insisting and doctor shopping, instead of getting the answers you are looking for, you'll get lots of unnecessary tests and even more things to worry about. Accept the reality that the medical system cannot give all the answers. Tests are not 100% accurate; good results are not a guarantee of either present or future well being, bad results can be false positive. Unexplained pains are the rule rather than exception. The medical system can usually rule out a few dangerous conditions. After that is done, stop testing and if not satisfied with the help you get, seek help outside of the traditional medical establishment.

Be aware that a good health insurance can predispose you to unnecessary procedures and tests. It gives a financial incentive for doctors to do more. In addition to that, curb your own sense of entitlement. The best use of health insurance in most cases is no use at all, provided you are feeling well and living a healthy lifestyle. Trying to get more things checked just to get full use of your insurance can cause you trouble. Pain as a result of greed or search for reassurance from the medical establishment is the usual outcome. When considering any test, try to find out how likely you are to have a condition that the test is testing for. If this likelihood is low, do not do the test because a positive (abnormal) result is much more likely to be false positive and you'll have to go through additional tests and procedures unnecessarily. In medical schools, students are taught to rule things out, "just to make sure" you don't have something. This is a harmful practice in addition to being expensive for those who end up paying for it—all of us in the end.

What can you do when you feel undertreated, overtreated, or mistreated? If you feel undertreated (your doctor is not addressing a bothersome symptom) because your doctor cannot discover what causes it, tell your doctor that you wish treatment in spite of the fact that a specific disease was not discovered, and ask about alternatives. The other option is just to accept to live with the symptom. Do not accept the implication that you are crazy, but consider the possibility of emotional and social discord in your life contributing to your symptom. On the other hand, if you feel your doctor is giving you too many pills, tell him that while you understand that he tries to follow guidelines, for you taking more isn't worth the trouble. Don't feel obliged to explain your reasons, but if you wish, you can mention the risks of interactions (these may come up unexpectedly with some medications when drinking grapefruit juice, taking medicine for a cold, or having some alcohol), side-effects, and the inconvenience of monitoring tests to name a few. Mistreatment can be decreased by active involvement of a family member with the care of a person who has lost capacity for decision making and cannot voice their objection.

How do you deal with being offered more and more pills for the same condition? Do not be too surprised if you are asked to take more and more pills over time, even if your condition hasn't gotten worse. As a result of the process called medicalization, what was considered normal not long ago may now be labeled a disease that requires treatment. This process may continue for a while. The Europeans and Canadians who have access to the same information do not follow this trend to the same degree, because the influence of the industry is not as strong. If you are told that, according to the new standard, you require medical treatment for something, take it with some humor. Following guidelines to the letter is sure to profit someone, but not sure to make you healthier and definitely won't make you immortal.

Cancer screening is not as useful as it may seem. Do not be fooled by screening campaigns even when they are led by truly well meaning people. The usefulness of cancer screening is questionable if you are at low risk for that cancer, with possible exception of triennial cervical cancer screening—Pap smear. Any reasonable physician should be able to tell you whether you are at high or low risk for developing cancer, and you can find out yourself. Prostate cancer screening is not helpful at all according to the data available as of now (October 2004), usefulness of breast cancer screening is highly questionable. Also, when offered a test, consider asking your doctor whether she would get the test himself in your situation, then observe how confident she is in responding. Check out the British [1] and Canadian [2] screening information it is a lot less aggressive and less misleading.

The capabilities of modern medicine are far less impressive than they may appear. This is as much true in the treatment of ear infections, as it is in the treatment of cancers. With the exception of several infrequent cancers, cancer survival has changed minimally over the past forty years. The vast majority of medical problems are healed by themselves. Even when it comes to cancers, active coping style, hopefulness, and awareness of the possibility of a spontaneous cure are, in my opinion, more important than belief in the "miracles" of modern medicine. While modern medicine can be helpful, a belief that it is the answer to deadly diseases leads to expectations that are bound to be disappointed, often with lost time and increased suffering.

---

[1] See http://ebm.bmjjournals.com/
[2] See http://www.ctfphc.org/

Understand how much benefit any risky treatment is likely to provide before consenting to it. If the benefit is small, even minor risks may not be worth it. Also, do not expose your expectations to your doctor or you're likely to get what you expect, even if it is harmful. Instead, listen first to what your doctor will offer, then ask his or her opinion about the tests or treatments that you had in mind, but without pressure. Usually you do not need more tests if a US trained doctor did not offer you more; we already do too many tests here. When it comes to surgical procedures, do not dismiss the risks, bad things can really happen. Do not make a final decision in a rush or before speaking with the surgeon who is going to operate on you. If you decide in advance, you may not be aware of all the risks. If the risks are not acceptable to you, explore non-surgical alternatives. If you are offered a risky treatment, inquire how much benefit it is likely to bring. Then make up your own mind about using it. The doctor, who cannot tell you about a measure of benefit, may simply be following an old habit that is not based on evidence.

Be proactive in managing your own or your family's end-of-life care. When caring for a family member who is old, very sick or terminally ill, do not expect that your doctor will initiate the movement away from intervention and more testing. The doctor will usually be afraid of being perceived as giving up and being uncaring with legal repercussions that can follow. Therefore it is the family's responsibility to initiate this with the doctor. Let go of your guilt: you are fooling yourself if you think that by doing more medical treatments you are doing more for the patient. Be prepared to make decisions in the face of uncertainty, because the medical system is unable to provide certainty. Waiting longer may never yield more clarity as to the patient's future. While some waiting time may be warranted, be prepared to decide in the moment. Indecision and inaction are usually equivalent to deciding to have more medical interventions.

The best care is not what is available but what is appropriate. When the time comes, being prepared to let go of a loved one provides for a more natural way of dying. Lack of medical care is not equivalent to lack of caring. Caring is not the same as curing or trying to cure. A dying person's needs are very few; most of the medical conditions need not be treated because treatments do not provide short term gain. Instead, palliative measures may be more appropriate. Consider a 'Do Not Hospitalize' directive in addition to 'Do Not Resuscitate' and 'Do Not Intubate' for a loved one dying at a nursing home. In some cases, 'No Intravenous Fluids' or 'No Artificial Nutrition and Hydration,' and 'No Antibiotics' are appropriate and necessary to decrease suffering. Do not be hesitant to sign those in advance; they don't indicate a lack of caring or giving up. Taking care of this will lower yours or your loved one's chances of dying in an intensive care unit with all sorts of tests done and devices attached to the person.

Excessive attachment to the physical brings additional suffering. It manifests itself, at the same time, as clinging to stay alive at any cost, and a belief that the high-technology of the medical system can overcome suffering and death. This attachment often results in a loss of dignity, as we cling to a machine and a pill in our last moments. To overcome this confusion and the unnecessary suffering caused by it, I believe, one needs to direct one's attention to a spiritual or philosophical direction, and withdraw the authority that one has given to the physical powers of medical care.

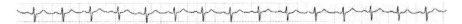

22 Afterword

I hope that I have succeeded laying out a more realistic view of the medical system. One can no longer simply assume that a figure of authority, such as a physician, will do what is best for his patient. Multiple conflicts of interest, some of which have existed for ages and others particular to the United States of end of 20th and beginning of 21st centuries, make it difficult for any doctor to be a true patient advocate. The health care system, or as I call it Health Care Machine, is becoming more mechanical with many decisions made without reflection or consideration of individual differences, but based on prevailing doctrine and predetermined algorithms. The health care industry is a business with enormous power and enormous influence, which extends to medical education, medical research, and health care policy. Many doctors acting within this system lose the ability of critical thought, since this ability is systematically taken away and discouraged by multiple mechanisms. Three factors more and more discourage any creative thought and tend to turn medical care into an assembly line type of process. These are the threat of a lawsuit, biased research and education, a trend of pre-determined medical protocols to treat various health conditions. The physician is usually unaware of gradually becoming a prisoner of the system and then automatically acting on its behalf, much like a robot.

An unintended but deleterious effect of the medical industry is to promote itself to the point when systematic exaggeration leads to creation of a false belief that medicine is something that it is not. Most cancer screening is of very limited value, and most cancers are just as incurable by the medical efforts now, as they were when they were first discovered. This illusion of medical omnipotence is played out to the extreme in dealing with the end-of-life processes, where most old people in the US are dying in hospitals, and many in the intensive care units after getting tests and procedures which have been shown to actually shorten their lives. Having delegated the decision-making to the doctors, who are inextricably intertwined with the rest of the system, our end-of-life care becomes a business decision as seen from the data that shows one determinant of the place of death—availability of hospital beds. We make a decision to surrender ourselves to the medical system because, without overtly stating so, the medical system fosters a belief that it can provide immortality (as for instance by its efforts in cloning). This then drives our medical decisions in everyday life and culminates at the time of dying.

Thus I turn my attention to death and the process of dying. While this may seem disheartening initially, when the true limits of medicine are realized and accepted, there is a possibility of more preparedness, clearer decision making, and peace of mind. Letting go of the faith in this system permits our release from the shackles that keep us clinging to high technology and induce suffering.

Life can be less dominated by the traps of big business. With the knowledge in this book, one is less likely to surrender to inhumane testing and procedures offered under the pretext of prolonging life. Such testing and procedures only add profit to the industry and suffering to the believers. I think it is a lot healthier for all patients, regardless how much or little education they may have, to adopt a belief that they are the authority when it comes to knowing what is good for them. As a physician, when I'm dealing with patients who are comfortable refusing what I offer, I know that these people are not likely to become victims of the system. They preserve their integrity by not putting me (and the institution of medical care) above themselves. They are more likely to live and die free.

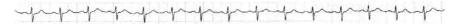

References

AAFP This Week (Vol. 5, No. 40) *Manufacturer Cancels Shipment of the Flu Vaccine.* Compiled by the AAFP News Department, 10/5/04.

Abeloff: Clinical Oncology, 3rd ed., Chapter 94 – *Cancer of the breast,* 2004 Elsevier.

Aboulker-Muscat, Colette. *Alone with the One.* ACMI press, 1995, New York.

ACC/AHA *2002 guideline update for the management of patients with chronic stable angina:* a report of the American College of Cardiology/American Heart Association Task Force on Practice Guidelines (Committee to Update the 1999 Guidelines for the Management of Patients With Chronic Stable Angina).

ACOG (American College of Obstetrics and Gynecology) News Release. *ACOG Issues State of the Art Guide to Hormone Therapy.* September 30, 2004. http://www.acog.com/from_home/publications/press_releases/nr09-30-04-2.cfm?printerF

ACOG Committee Opinion: Committee on obstetric practice: Down's syndrome screening: 1994; No. 141 (Replaces No. 76, 1989).

Agra Y; Pelayo M; Sacristan M; Sacristán A; Serra C; Bonfill X., *Chemotherapy versus best supportive care for extensive small cell lung cancer.* The Cochrane Database of Systematic Reviews. This Cochrane Review is unmodified this issue. Review first published in Issue 4, 2003.

American Academy of Family Physicians. *Summary of Policy Recommendations for the Periodic Health Examination.* Kansas City, MO, Authors, 1999b.

Anonymous. A controlled trial to improve care for seriously ill hospitalized patients: The Study to Understand Prognoses and Preferences for Outcomes and Risks of Treatments (SUPPORT). JAMA. 1995;274:1591-1598.

Antsaklis, A. Papantoniou, N, Xigakis, A, et al. *Genetic amniocentesis in women 20-34 years old: associated risk.* Prenat Diagn 2000; 20:247.

Barnholtz-Sloan JS; Severson RK; Vaishampayan U; Hussain M., Survival analysis of distant prostate cancer by decade (1973-1997) in

the Detroit Metropolitan Surveillance, Epidemiology and End Results (SEER) Program registry: has outcome improved? (United
States). Cancer causes & control : CCC [Cancer Causes Control]
2003 Sep; 14 (7), pp. 681-5.

Bath PMW; Bath FJ; Smithard DG. *Interventions for dysphagia in acute
stroke.* The Cochrane Database of Systematic Reviews. Issue 4,
1999.

Belch JJF et al. *Critical issues in peripheral arterial disease detection and management: A Call to Action.* Arch Intern Med 2003; 163: 884-92.
Abstracted in The Family Practice Newsletter Vol 19, No 1, Jan 1;
2003.

Benn, P. Improved antenatal screening for Down's syndrome. Lancet
2003; 361: 794.

Canadian Cancer Society. *Five-year relative cancer survival in Canada, 1992.*
Special topic from Canadian Cancer Statistics 2002. Available at
http://www.cancer.ca/ccs/internet/standard/0,3182,3172_367655
_39066503_langId-en,00.html

CDC/NCHS, National Vital Statistics System.

Chiasson JL, Josse RG, Gomis R, et al. *Acarbose for prevention of type 2
diabetes mellitus: the STOP-NIDDM randomised trial. Lancet*
2002;359:2072-7.
http://www.ncbi.nlm.nih.gov/entrez/query.fcgi?cmd=Retrieve&d
b=PubMed&list_uids=12086760&dopt=Abstract

Clegg A, Scott D A, Sidhu M, Hewitson P, Waugh N, A rapid and systematic review of the clinical effectiveness and cost-effectiveness of
paclitaxel, docetaxel, gemcitabine and vinorelbine in non-small-cell
lung cancer. Health Technology Assessment; 2001; v. 5(no. 32), p1,
(1-195)

Cochrane Review on Screening for Breast Cancer with Mammography. By: Olsen,
Ole, Gotzsche, Peter C, Lancet, 0099-5355, October 20, 2001, Vol.
358, Issue 9290

Coffield, Ashley B. MPH, et al *Priorities Among Recommended Clinical Preventive Services.* American Journal of Preventive Medicine 2001;21(1).

Coldman AJ, Phillips N. Pickles TA. *Trends in prostate cancer incidence and mortality: an analysis of mortality change by screening intensity.* CMAJ Canadian Medical Association Journal. 168(1):31-5, 2003 Jan 7.

Coull BM, et al. Anticoagulants and antiplatelet agents in acute ischemic *stroke*: report of the Joint *Stroke* Guideline Development Committee of the American Academy of Neurology and the American *Stroke* Association (a division of the American Heart Association). Neurology 2002 Jul 9;59.

Diabetes Prevention Program Research Group. *Reduction in the incidence of type 2 diabetes with lifestyle intervention or metformin.* N Engl J Med 2002;346:393-403.

Ellestad, Stuart RJ, MH: National survey of exercise stress testing facilities. Chest 77:94, 1980.

Elmore, Joann G et al. *Ten-Year Risk of False Positive Screening Mammograms and Clinical Breast Examinations.* The New England Journal of Medicine. V338(16) 16 April 1998 pp 1089-1096.

Epstein, Gerald N., M.D. *Healing Visualizations.* Bantam New Age Books 1999.

Epstein,Gerald N. M.D. web site http://www.drgerryepstein.org/light/wisdom0406.html.

Etzioni R; Penson DF; Legler JM; di Tommaso D; Boer R; Gann PH; Feuer EJ., *Overdiagnosis due to prostate-specific antigen screening: lessons from U.S. prostate cancer incidence trends.* Journal of the National Cancer Institute [J Natl Cancer Inst] 2002 Jul 3; 94 (13), pp. 981-90.

Faller, Hermann M.D., Ph.D.; Bülzebruck, Heinrich Ph.D. *Coping and Survival in Lung Cancer: A 10-Year Follow-Up.* American Journal of Psychiatry. Vol 159(12), Dec 2002 p 2105–2107.

Gabbe: Obstetrics - *Normal and Problem Pregnancies*, 4th ed., Chapter 16 – Malpresentations, 2002 Churchill Livingstone, Inc.

Gifford, Deidre Spelliscy MD, MPH et al. *A meta-analysis of infant outcomes after breach delivery.* Obstetrics and Gynecology 1995;85:1047-54.

Goff BA, et al, *Frequency of symptoms of ovarian cancer in women presenting to primary care clinics.* JAMA 2004; 291: 2705-12. Abstracted in The Family Practice Newsletter Vol. 20, No. 15, July 15, 2004.

Grimes, David A. MD; Lobo, Rogerio A. MD *Perspectives on the Women's Health Initiative Trial of Hormone Replacement Therapy;* Obstetrics & Gynecology, Vol. 100(6), December 2002, p 1344–1353.

Groopman, Jerome E, MD., *The Thirty Years' War.* The New Yorker, June 4, 2001, p.32.

Groopman, Jerome, MD., *The Anatomy of Hope*, Random House, NY, 2003; New York Times Book Review, Sunday, Feb 22, 2004, p.22. Abstracted in The Family Practice Newsletter Vol. 20 No. 11, 2004.

Grundy SM, Cleeman JI, Merz CN, et al. *Implications of recent clinical trials for the National Cholesterol Education Program Adult Treatment Panel III guidelines. Circulation* 2004;110:227-39. Abstracted in Prescriber's Letter Vol. 11, No. 8, August 2004.

Ho PM. et al, *Predictors of cognitive decline following coronary artery bypass graft surgery.* Annals of Thoracic Surgery. 77(2):597-603; discussion 603, 2004 Feb.

Hofmann, Jan C. MD et al. *Patient Preferences for Communication with Physicians about End-of-Life Decisions.* Annals of Intern Med, 1 July 1997, Vol. 127, Issue 1, pp. 1-12.

Hollander, Jay B. M.D. Ananias C. Diokno M.D. Chapter 48 - *Prostate Gland Disease.* Duthie: Practice of Geriatrics, 3rd ed., 1998 W. B. Saunders Company.

Hunt JO. et al, *Quality of life 12 months after coronary artery bypass graft surgery.* Heart & Lung: Journal of Acute & Critical Care. 29(6):401-11, 2000 Nov-Dec.

JNC-VII. Seventh Report of the Joint National Committee on Prevention, Detection, Evaluation, and Treatment of High Blood Pressure 2003.

Katsura H. et al, [*Outcome of repeated pulmonary aspiration in frail elderly. The Project Team for Aspiration Pneumonia*]. Nippon Ronen Igakkai Zasshi - Japanese Journal of Geriatrics. 35(5):363-6, 1998 May.

Kerlikowske K et al., Positive predictive value of screening mammography by age and family history of breast cancer. JAMA 1993 Nov 24; 270:2444-2450. Abstracted in Journal Watch December 10, 1993.

Knipp SC et al., Evaluation of brain injury after coronary artery bypass grafting. A prospective study using neuropsychological assessment and diffusion-weighted magnetic resonance imaging. European Journal of Cardio-Thoracic Surgery. 25(5):791-800, 2004 May.

Kolata, Gina, *New Studies Question Value of Opening Arteries.* The New York Times Magazine, March 21, 2004.

Kopes-Kerr, Colin P. M.D. M.P.H. Editor. The Family Practice Newsletter Vol. 20 No. 11, 2004.

Kopes-Kerr, Colin P. M.D. *My colon cancer dilemma.* The Family Practice Newsletter Vol.20 No.13 July 2004.

Kumar: Robbins and Cotran: *Pathologic Basis of Disease*, 7th ed. 2005 Elsevier.

Makinen T. et al. *Family history and prostate cancer screening with prostate-specific antigen.* Journal of Clinical Oncology. 20(11):2658-63, 2002 Jun 1.

Martz, William D., MD. *How to Boost Your Bottom Line With an Office Procedure.* Family Practice Management - November/December 2003.

Mayo Clinic heart center from www.mayoclinic.com June 28, 2004.

MedlinePlus, a service of the US National Library of Medicine and The National institute of health.

Meier, Diane E. M.D. R. Sean Morrison M.D. Judith C. Ahronheim M.D. Chapter 12 - *Palliative Care.* Duthie: Practice of Geriatrics, 3rd ed., 1998 W. B. Saunders Company.

Melnikow J, Nuovo J, Willan AR et al. *Natural history of cervical squamous intraepithelial lesions: a meta-analysis.* Ob Gyn 1998; 92, 727-35, abstracted in The Family Practice Newsletter Vol. 14, No. 4, Feb 15, 1999.

Mesa García A; Pérez García FJ., [*Survival in prostatic cancer, treated conservatively*]. Actas urologicas espanolas [Actas Urol Esp] 2000 Jun; 24 (6), pp. 475-80.

Molassiotis A. et al. Symptom distress, coping style and biological variables as predictors of survival after bone marrow transplantation. Journal of Psychosomatic Research. 42(3):275-85, 1997 Mar.

Montagnini, Marcos L., MD, FACP, Mary E. Moat, RN, MS, BC, CHPN; *Non–pain symptom management in palliative care*. Clinics in Family Practice. Volume 6 • Number 2 • June 2004 W. B. Saunders Company.

Murray & Nadel: Textbook of Respiratory Medicine, 3rd ed., 2000 W. B. Saunders Company.

National Cancer Institute Monograph 44, *Conference on Spontaneous Regression of Cancer*. November 1976. DHEW Publication No. (NIH) 76-1038.

NHS Breast Screening Programme Publication No 54:*Review of radiation risk in breast screening*. February 2003 (Sheffield: NHS Cancer Screening Programmes) ISBN 1-871997-99-2.

Noble: Textbook of Primary Care Medicine, 3rd ed., 2001 Mosby, Inc.

Nyström L et al. *Long-term effects of mammography screening: Updated overview of the Swedish randomized trials*. Lancet 2002 Mar 16; 359:909-19. Abstracted in Journal Watch Women's Health May 8, 2002.

O'Mathúna, Dónal P. PhD *The Placebo Effect and Alternative Therapies*. Alternative Medicine Alert Published: June 01, 2003.

Odibo, Anthony O; Macones, George A. *Current concepts regarding vaginal birth after cesarean delivery*. Current Opinion in Obstetrics and Gynecology. Vol 15(6), Dec 2003, pp 479-482.

Okie, Susan. Missing Data on Celebrex. *Full Study Altered Picture of Drug*. Washington Post, Sunday, August 5, 2001; Page A11.

Ottesen GL. Carcinoma in situ of the female breast. A clinicopathological, immunohistological, and DNA ploidy study. APMIS. Supplementum. (108):1-67, 2003.

Pedtgrella JR et al., Effects of hyaluronate sodium on pain and physical functioning in osteoarthritis of the knee: A randomized, double-blind, placebo-controlled clinical trial. Arch Intern Med 2002; 162: 292-8. Felson DT, Anderson JJ, Hyaluronate sodium injections for osteoarthritis: Hope, hype, and hard truth. Arch Intern Med 2002; 163: 245-7. Abstracted in Action Advisor for Primary Care, March 2002.

Prescriber's Letter, Lots of drug study results are being disseminated with a favorable spin. May 2004, Vol. 11.

Prescriber's Letter. *HHS, ADA warn Americans of "Pre-diabetes," Encourages people to take healthy steps to reduce risks.* Therapeutic Research Center. Pharmacist's Letter/Prescriber's Letter 2002;18:180421.

Prescriber's Letter. *Statistics.* October 2004; Vol: 11, No. 10.

Pritchard RS, Fisher ES, Teno JM, Sharp SM, Reding DJ, Knaus WA, Wennberg JE, Lynn J. Influence of patient preferences and local health system characteristics on the place of death. J Am Geriatr Soc. 1998;46:1242-1250.

Randolph WM et al. Regular mammography use is associated with elimination of age-related disparities in size and stage of breast cancer at diagnosis. Ann Intern Med 2002 Nov 19; 137:783-90. Abstracted in Journal Watch December 31, 2002.

Ray WA et al. *Oral erythromycin and the risk of sudden death from cardiac causes.* N Engl J Med 2004 Sep 9; 351: 1089-96. Abstracted in Journal Watch Vol. 24, No. 20 Oct 15, 2004.

Reuter M. et al. [*High-resolution computed tomography of the lungs in pediatric patients*].[erratum appears in Rofo Fortschr Geb Rontgenstr Neuen Bildgeb Verfahr 2002 Sep;174(9):1179]. [Review] [85 refs] [German] ROFO-Fortschritte auf dem Gebiet der Rontgenstrahlen und der Bildgebenden V. 174(6):684-95, 2002 Jun.

Ries LAG, Kosary CL, Hankey BF, et al. (eds). *SEER Cancer Statistics Review, 1973-1995. Bethesda, MD:* National Cancer Institute, 1998. Adapted, from Murray & Nadel, 2000.

Rinpoche, Sogyal, *The Tibetan Book of Living and Dying.* Publisher: HarperSanFrancisco 1993.

Robbins Pathologic Basis of Disease, 7th ed., 2004 Elsevier p. 176.

Sahl P et al. Incidence of breast cancer in Norway and Sweden during the introduction of nationwide screening: prospective cohort study. BMJ 2004; 328: 921-4. Abstracted in Action Advisor for primary care Vol.6 No.8. August 2004.

Schwartz LM et al. *Enthusiasm for cancer screening in the United States.* JAMA 2004; 291: 71-8. Abstracted in The Family Practice Newsletter Vol. 20 No. 11, 2004.

SEER Program, National Cancer Institute, *Cancer Survival Rates*, publicly available at http://seer.cancer.gov/publications

Shuster M et al. Prospective evaluation of clinical assessment in the diagnosis and treatment of clavicle fracture: Are radiographs really necessary? Can J Emerg Med 2003; 4: 309; reviewed in Action Advisor for Primary Care Vol. 6 No. 8, August 2004.

Siegel, Bernie, MD. Love, Medicine and Miracles. 1986. Harper & Row Publish Inc.

Silverstein FE. Et. Al. Gastrointestinal toxicity with celecoxib vs non-steroidal anti-inflammatory drugs for osteoarthritis and rheumatoid arthritis: the CLASS study: A randomized controlled trial. Celecoxib Long-term Arthritis Safety Study. JAMA. 284(10):1247-55, 2000 Sep 13.

Skowronski DM, et al. *Oculo-respiratory syndrome: A new vaccine-associated adverse event?* Clin Infect Dis 2003; 36, 705-13; abstracted in The Family Practice Newsletter V19, N1, Jan1, 2003.

Smith GCS et al. *Caesarean section and risk of unexplained stillbirth in subsequent pregnancy.* Lancet 2003 Nov 29; 362:1779-84. Abstracted in Journal Watch Women's Health Feb 11, 2004.

Stewart SL; King JB; Thompson TD; Friedman C; Wingo PA, *Cancer mortality surveillance—United States, 1990-2000.* MMWR. Surveillance summaries : Morbidity and mortality weekly report. Surveillance summaries [MMWR Surveill Summ] 2004 Jun 4; 53 (3), pp. 1-108.

Sutherland CM; Mather FJ., Long-term survival and prognostic factors in patients with regional breast cancer (skin, muscle, and/or chest wall attachment). Cancer [Cancer] 1985 Mar 15; 55 (6), pp. 1389-97.

Sutherland CM; Mather FJ., Long-term survival and prognostic factors in breast cancer patients with localized (no skin, muscle, or chest wall attachment) disease with and without positive lymph nodes. Cancer [Cancer] 1986 Feb 1; 57 (3), pp. 622-9.

The Dartmouth Atlas of Health Care 1999. Center for the Evaluative Clinical Sciences at Dartmouth Medical School. www.dartmouthatlas.org/about.php. 1999. *Overuse and Underuse of End of Life Care*. Chapter 7, The Quality of Medical Care in the United States. Section Thirteen.

The Economist. Science and technology. *The future of cancer treatment up close, and personal.* Oct 16, 2004.

The Medical Letter Vol 46, August 30, 2004.

Tinetti, Mary E. MD, Terry Fried, MD. *The End of the Disease Era.* The American Journal of Medicine, February 1, 2004 Vol 116, pp. 179-185.

Topol EJ, Falk GW. *A coxib a day won't keep the doctor away.* Lancet 2004; 364: 639-40. Abstracted in Action Advisor for Primary Care Vol. 6 No. 8 August 2004.

Tracy, Thomas F. Jr, MD; Crawford, Linda S. JD; Krizek, Thomas J. MD; Kern, Kenneth A. MD, *When Medical Error Becomes Medical Malpractice: The Victims and the Circumstances.* Archives of Surgery, The New England Surgical Society, Vol 138(4), April 2003, p 447–454.

Treatment Guidelines from The Medical Letter, Vol. 2 (Issue 22), June 2004.

Truog, Robert D., MD et al. *Recommendations for end-of-life care in the intensive care unit: The Ethics Committee of the Society of Critical Care Medicine.* Critical Care Medicine. Volume 29, Number 12, December 2001, Copyright © 2001 Lippincott Williams & Wilkins.

United States Preventive Services Task Force. *Screening for cervical cancer: Recommendations and rationale.* Accessed February 6, 2003, at http://www.ahrq.gov/clinic/3rduspstf/cervcan/cervcanrr.htm and http://www.ahrq.gov/clinic/3rduspstf/cervcan/cervcanrr2.htm.

United States Preventive Services Task Force. *Screening for Prostate Cancer: Recommendations and Rationale.* Originally in Ann Intern Med 2002;137:915-6. Agency for Healthcare Research and Quality,

Rockville, MD.
http://www.ahrq.gov/clinic/3rduspstf/prostatescr/prostaterr.htm.

United States Preventive Services Task Force. USPSTF recommendation: *Screening for Breast Cancer.* February 2002.
http://www.ahrq.gov/clinic/3rduspstf/breastcancer/

United States Preventive Services Task Force: Guide to Clinical Preventive Services. *Screening for Iron Deficiency Anemia.* Baltimore, MD, Williams & Wilkins, 1996.

Venning P. et al. Randomised controlled trial comparing cost effectiveness of general practitioners and nurse practitioners in primary care. BMJ. 320(7241):1048-53, 2000 Apr 15.

Welch HG; Schwartz LM; Woloshin S., *Are increasing 5-year survival rates evidence of success against cancer?* JAMA : the journal of the American Medical Association [JAMA] 2000 Jun 14; 283 (22), pp. 2975-8.

Wennberg, John E et al. Use of hospitals, physician visits, and hospice care during last six months of life among cohorts loyal to highly respected hospitals in the United States. BMJ 2004;
328:607 (13 March), doi:10.1136/bmj.328.7440.607.

Wiebelt H; Hakulinen T; Ziegler H; Stegmaier C., [Do cancer patients survive longer today than before? Survival analysis of cancer patients in the Saar region from 1972 to 1986]. Sozial- und Praventivmedizin [Soz Praventivmed] 1991; 36 (2), pp. 86-95.

Index

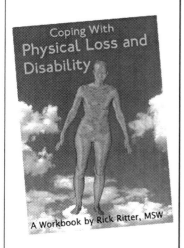

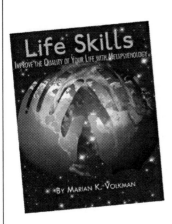

Exclusive offer for readers of *Secrets of Medical Decision Making*

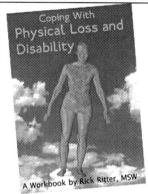 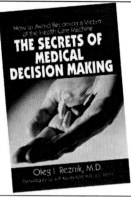 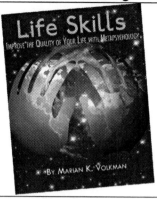

Share the power of Loving Healing Press Books

Order direct from the publisher with this form and save!

Order Form – 15% Discount Off List Price!

Ship To:

_____
Name

_____
Address

_____
Address

_____ _____
City   State

_____
District   Country   Zip/Post code

_____
Daytime phone #

_____
email address

_____ _____/_____
Card #   Expires

_____
                    Signature

Secrets of Med. Dec. ____ x $16 = _____

Coping w/Phys. Loss ____ x $15 = _____

Life Skills by MKV ___ x $14.50 = _____

Subtotal = _____

Residents of Michigan: 6% tax = _____

Shipping charge (see below) _____

Your Total _$_____

Shipping price per copy via:
☐ Priority Mail (+ $3.50) ☐ Int'l Airmail (+ $4) ☐ USA MediaMail/4th Class (+ $2)

Fax Order Form back to (734)663-6861 or
Mail to LHP, 5145 Pontiac Trail, Ann Arbor, MI 48105

LaVergne, TN USA
14 September 2010
196874LV00001B/17/A